classic /Historical

Bureau of Hospital Administration, Research Series No. 1

PROBABILITY SAMPLING
OF HOSPITALS AND PATIENTS

IRENE HESS
Survey Research Center

DONALD C. RIEDEL
Bureau of Hospital Administration

THOMAS B. FITZPATRICK
Bureau of Hospital Administration

The University of Michigan, Ann Arbor, 1961

Foreword

This monograph is a direct outgrowth of an extensive study, entitled *Study of Hospital and Medical Economics,* which was undertaken at The University of Michigan at the request of a Governor's Study Commission. In the design of that study, it was necessary to find a way to obtain from a manageable number of institutions data that could be generalized to the state as a whole or sacrifice the scope and depth of various facets of the study in attempting to deal directly with the entire universe. The resultant method is a ranking contribution which grew out of the practical necessities of a major research effort.

The authors have used the techniques developed during the initial stages of the *Study of Hospital and Medical Economics* as a point of departure to discuss in some depth how probability sampling can be applied to hospitals and patients in general. The result should be of great value to the field of hospital and medical economics where there are numerous opportunities for profitable application.

The monograph is essentially the product of the Bureau of Hospital Administration, although considerable cooperation from the Survey Research Center was involved. Irene Hess, A.B., was responsible primarily for the design and selection of the hospital samples described, and Donald C. Riedel, Ph.D., and Thomas B. Fitzpatrick, M.S., for the sampling of patients and data collection. The three worked closely on preparation of the manuscript.

The Bureau of Hospital Administration is pleased to offer this as the first of a series of monographs that will bear on substantive and methodological problems in the field of hospital and medical economics.

A large share of the work done was made possible by the generous support of The W. K. Kellogg Foundation.

Walter J. McNerney
Director
Bureau of Hospital Administration

Preface

This monograph is designed to satisfy several objectives: to focus attention on controlled selection as a useful technique in probability sampling when a relatively small sample of hospitals is desired; to contribute, through detailed description of selection procedures, to the understanding and interpretation of the Michigan study, as well as to share this experience in probability sampling of hospitals and patients with investigators interested in conducting similar research; to make data on sampling variability available to others for purposes of sample design; to demonstrate to persons responsible for research in the field of hospital and medical care that probability sampling is practicable and fruitful, as illustrated by empirical results from the Michigan study.

Because of these distinct but related objectives, the individual reader may not find all segments of this monograph of equal interest. For example, the general discussion of sampling presented in Chapter II contains nothing new to the sampling statistician, and the mathematical formulas related to sampling variability in Chapter V may not be immediately comprehensible to the hospital administrator who has no background in statistics.

Many persons made significant contributions in the planning and analysis stages of the study, and to the preparation of the manuscript. Dr. Rensis Likert, Director of the Institute for Social Research and member of the Advisory Committee for the *Study of Hospital and Medical Economics,* first recommended a probability sample of hospitals. The authors also acknowledge the suggestions and helpful criticism offered by Walter J. McNerney, Director of the *Study of Hospital and Medical Economics;* Kenton E. Winter, Research Associate, Bureau of Public Health Economics; and Mrs. Betty Tableman, Administrative Analyst, Division of Hospital and Medical Facilities, Michigan Department of Health.

A large volume of data had to be programmed and tabulated. Of particular help were Dr. Robert C. F. Bartels, Director of the Computing Center of The University; Robert J. Koch, Frederick J. Marshall, and Alfred R. Keller of the Michigan Hospital Service; and John A. Sonquist and his staff of the Statistical Analysis Section of the Institute for Social Research.

Miss Jean Harter, Administrative Assistant, Sampling Section of the Survey Research Center, and Mrs. Mary B. Woolfenden, Research Associate, Bureau of Hospital Administration, were helpful in the controlled selection of hospitals and in the data coding phases of the study, respectively. Mrs. Doris Royster and Miss Katherine L. Gentner deserve special acknowledgment for their fortitude in typing the many drafts of the manuscript.

A number of persons read the monograph in various stages of completion and made suggestions for its improvement: from the Sampling Section of the Survey Research Center, Dr. Leslie Kish, Head, and N. Krishnan Namboodiri and R. Krishna Pillai, Research Assistants; from the Bureau of Hospital Administration, Symond R. Gottlieb, Gary G. Grenholm, John R. Griffith, Lawrence A. Hill, Henry J. Morris, and Dr. Grover C. Wirick, Jr. Responsibility for any shortcomings of the sample design, analysis, or reporting, however, must rest with the authors.

Finally, the authors acknowledge the cooperation of the hospitals and physicians of Michigan who were selected in the sample. With the exception of one hospital which was undergoing extensive remodeling at the time of the study, the hospitals contributed data and often clerical help without reservation. Over ninety-nine per cent of the physicians contacted agreed to be interviewed. This demonstration of interest and willingness to help should not pass unnoticed.

I. H.
D. C. R.
T. B. F.

Ann Arbor
June, 1961

Table of Contents

V. SAMPLING VARIABILITY

List of Illustrations and Figures

List of Tables

Chapter I

Introduction

The *Study of Hospital and Medical Economics*, a major research endeavor recently completed by the Bureau of Hospital Administration, The University of Michigan, was undertaken at the behest of a Governor's Study Commission appointed to inquire into circumstances surrounding increased rates of prepayment of hospital and medical care costs. The general purposes of the study were: (1) to look at the health needs, the consumption of health services, and the health expenditures of the Michigan population; (2) to inventory, characterize, and evaluate purveyors of health services; (3) to examine critically the insurance, prepayment, and other mechanisms designed to bring the people and the purveyors together; and (4) to identify existing controls in the voluntary system of provision of and payment for health care. Thirteen individual projects were carried out under these general purposes. The projects varied greatly in scope, depth, and purpose; but each had its place in the over-all pattern. Briefly, they were:

1. The General Population of the State
    a) "Population Survey." A study of a cross-section sample of the Michigan population with regard to its consumption of and expenditures for health services; its insurance coverage and other resources; its unmet health needs and attitudes toward early care.

2. The Providers of Care
    a) "Character and Effectiveness of Hospital Use." A study of the hospitalized population, various measures of its use of hospitals, and evaluation of the effectiveness with which the hospital was used by patients with selected diagnoses.
    b) "Changing Patterns of Care." A pilot study of the impact of advances in medical science on hospital care as seen in changing patterns of patient care in selected diagnoses for the years 1938, 1948, and 1958.
    c) "An Inventory of Health Manpower." A count of physicians, dentists, nurses, and members of other health professions and occupations, with some speculation on adequacy of supply and on methods of increasing the supply.

   d) "Study of Accounting and Finance." An analysis of institu-
      tional accounting systems in terms of agreement with accepted
      standards of good hospital and general accounting practices.
      This study covered such factors as accounting, internal con-
      trols, budgets, cost analysis, and Blue Cross reimbursement of
      hospitals.
   e) "A Study of Hospitals and Allied Institutions." An inventory
      and multifaceted description of health facilities, and an anal-
      ysis of hospital costs and related factors.

3. Mechanisms of Payment for Health Services
   a) "Characteristics of Prepayment and Insurance Organizations
      and Their Coverages." An analysis of current prepayment and
      insurance benefits available to the population from the chief
      health insurers in Michigan, and a study of the actuarial and
      financial implications of the operations of health insurers and
      prepayers.
   b) "Experience and Community Rating." A study of groups who
      had switched from Blue Cross to private voluntary health in-
      surance, and vice versa, to determine whether or not there is
      any selection among these groups on the basis of loss ratios.
   c) "Effect of Group Characteristics on Claim Experience." A
      study designed to determine whether the claim experience of a
      group is affected by size of group, principal occupation, and
      geographic area.
   d) "A Study of the Relationship Between Levels of Benefits and
      Hospital Utilization." A study of how the available plan bene-
      fits influence the use of health services, as reflected in the ex-
      periences of two pairs of matched groups.
   e) "Effect of Layoffs on Continuity of Coverage and on Claim
      Experience." A study of the impact of recession and unemploy-
      ment on prepayment plans.
   f) "The Role of the Government in Personal Health Care." A
      description of the character and volume of government (fed-
      eral, state, local) payment for health services.

4. Controls
   a) "Controls Within and Upon the Voluntary Health System."
      An assessment of the use and effectiveness of the control mech-
      anisms in the voluntary system which govern quantity, quality
      and cost of health services.

For one of these studies, the "Character and Effectiveness of Hospital
Use," it was deemed essential to select a probability sample of hospitals
in Michigan, and, within each, to select a probability sample of patients.
Broadly construed, this study had three major objectives:

1. to describe the population of patients discharged from Michigan hospitals;

2. to ascertain how Michigan hospitals are being used; and

3. to determine the effectiveness of the use of Michigan hospitals.

For the first two objectives it was desirable to generalize to the entire hospitalized population of Michigan, including those patients discharged from both general and special institutions. Descriptive data and measures of hospital use would be most useful if this generalization were possible. Measurement of the effectiveness of hospital use was confined to general hospitals only.[1] Here it was important to be able to generalize to all general hospitals. For any one of these objectives, to sample the patients discharged from the universe of Michigan hospitals would have been of prohibitive expense.

Three of the other studies besides the "Character and Effectiveness of Hospital Use" were concerned with hospitals as institutions. Therefore, it was practical to design a sample to meet the needs of the four studies. This was accomplished by selecting a basic sample which could be expanded or subsampled as required. The sample consisted of 47 general hospitals. Two of the studies used this basic sample, one used an expanded sample of 88 hospitals, and the fourth study used a reduced sample of 33 hospitals. Although two of the studies included samples of special as well as general hospitals, only the basic sampling of general hospitals is discussed in this monograph, with particular reference to the study of the "Character and Effectiveness of Hospital Use."

Within the 47 hospitals, a probability sampling of discharges during 1958 was carried out in such a way as to represent all discharges from general hospitals in the state. On this sample of patients, demographic, diagnostic, and financial data were collected to describe the hospitalized population and to yield broad patterns of hospital use.

Variations in hospital use were measured in association with a number of variables descriptive of the patient, his physician, his hospital, and the source of payment of his hospital bill. In short, variations in use were measured against variations in other factors in order to identify significant influences on hospital utilization. If this analysis were to reveal extreme variation in patterns of hospital use within or between heterogeneous collectivities of patients, it could be argued that the variation was to be expected because of the heterogeneity itself. If, on the other hand, extreme variation persisted when enough variables were controlled to insure homogeneity of the patient groups compared, then a suspicion of ineffective use would be aroused. In other words, the use at the high end

---

[1] There were several important reasons for conducting the effectiveness study in general hospitals only. For a complete discussion of the concept and measurement of effectiveness, the interested reader is referred to the study report [11].

of the range might be overuse of the hospital; the use at the low end of the range might be underuse. Definitive evidence, however, would be lacking.

Therefore, on the hypothesis that influence of individual factors on effectiveness of hospital use could be ascertained adequately only if all major influences were identified and measured, it was deemed necessary to obtain all relevant details of a patient's disorder, study, and treatment, and to assess those with reference to other facts about him, his physician, and his hospital.

In broad terms, the first step was to establish standards of effective hospital use; the second, to measure deviations from the standards; and finally, to seek medical or extra-medical explanations of the deviations. Assumptions were that a patient's hospital medical record could be used for this purpose and that the attending physician's knowledge of the case, learned through personal interview, would yield additional medical information as well as extra-medical influences where these existed.

Anticipating that it would be impractical to study intensively the patterns of care in all diagnoses, subselection was decided upon. Using data compiled by the Commission on Professional and Hospital Activities, the sixty most common diagnoses which had appeared during the previous year in certain Michigan hospitals were examined.[2] Eighteen of these diagnoses were selected because of their high frequency and their representation of general and specialty practice and of medical and surgical conditions.

For these diagnoses, the determination of optimum effective care in Michigan hospitals—in effect, the establishment of standards—was entrusted to panels of specialists in various branches of medicine and surgery who developed criteria for appropriate hospital use, including indications for appropriate admission, appropriate length of stay, and appropriate procedures, taking into account various extenuating circumstances.

Aside from questions of sampling, successive steps in the study were:

1. Eighteen diagnoses were selected for intensive study.

2. Criteria of effectiveness of hospital use for each diagnosis were drawn up by panels of appropriate medical specialists.

3. Cases to be studied were selected as part of, and at the same time as, the over-all sample used for the description of the hospitalized population and the character of hospital use.

4. Field teams obtained the basic descriptive information for all cases in the over-all sample.

---

[2] The Commission on Professional and Hospital Activities, Ann Arbor, Michigan, is headed by Virgil N. Slee, M.D. Dr. Slee and his associates conduct a national program to collect centrally, analyze, and report data for member hospitals and their medical staffs.

5. Clinical abstracts were made from the medical records of selected cases within the 18 diagnoses, using standard forms for each diagnosis.

6. These abstracts were evaluated by physicians in the light of the established criteria. Cases were classified as to the appropriateness of the hospital admission, the length of stay, and the procedures received.

7. Interviews were held with the attending physicians of all cases who did not meet the criteria for admission or length of stay, and for a sample of those who did.
   a) Medical information beyond that available in the medical record was sought from the attending physician.
   b) Information on any other factors—economic, social, emotional, organizational—which might have affected the admission, length of stay, or procedures was also sought.
   c) In addition, the physician was asked his opinion about the effect of insurance on hospital use.

8. With the help of the interview material, a final evaluation of effectiveness was made.

The initial field work of the study was accomplished by two teams working in different areas of the state. Each team consisted of four senior medical students, one graduate physician, and one or more statistical clerks. In the field, determination of primary diagnosis was made by the medical student under the supervision of and with the assistance of the graduate physician. Preliminary and final evaluations were made by staff physicians, who also evaluated the interviews with the attending physicians of patients selected in the sample.

By re-examining the objectives of the study of the "Character and Effectiveness of Hospital Use," it may be seen more clearly that the description of the hospitalized population and the measurement of hospital use would have lost a great deal of meaning and usefulness if generalizations with reference to patient characteristics and patterns of utilization could not have been made to the entire population of hospital discharges in 1958. Moreover, since the subject of overuse and underuse of hospital facilities is a matter of wide interest and even controversy, conclusions must be solidly founded to gain credence. Therefore, the proper selection of a probability sample of hospitals and the selection of a probability sample of discharges within each hospital were major considerations in that study.

The application of probability sampling to general hospitals and patients is the major theme of this monograph.

Chapter II is devoted to a general discussion of sampling techniques used in the hospital and medical care field and to an exploration of specific types of sampling.

In Chapter III the sample design for the Michigan study is described and the controlled selection of general hospitals is presented. There follows a discussion of techniques employed to sample hospital records.

Chapter IV describes estimation procedures applicable to a sample of patients from general hospitals and to a sample of hospitals as institutions.

Chapter V presents techniques for estimating sampling variability, and gives selected findings from the study of the "Character and Effectiveness of Hospital Use." Some validation of sample data is offered through comparisons with estimates from independent sources. Probable sources of sampling variability are suggested, and design research recommended.

Chapter VI summarizes this experience in probability sampling, presents conclusions as to the practicability of the sampling techniques, and assesses the implications for future sampling research in the hospital and medical care field.

Chapter II

Sampling in the Hospital and Medical Care Field

The condition giving rise to sampling in the hospital and medical care field is essentially the same as that which has led to the use of sampling in other branches of social research—a desire for knowledge about a universe so large or dispersed that it is generally impracticable and frequently impossible to enumerate or contact each element in it. Recognition of the need for well-chosen samples has not resulted in immediate and widespread use of modern probability techniques. The situation can be attributed both to an undersupply of sampling technicians and to investigators who employ sampling practices of questionable merit.

It is the purpose of this chapter to survey some of the sampling methods used in medical care research, to describe several types of probability samples, and to supply minimum technical material to prepare readers with basic concepts necessary for the discussion of Chapter III, devoted to the Michigan experience in probability sampling of hospitals and patients.

SAMPLING PRACTICES IN CURRENT USE

To delimit the subject, only samples constructed for the purpose of estimating characteristics of some universe are considered. Sampling methods commonly used for this purpose are of two broad classes: probability samples, and nonprobability samples. A third class, defined as a 100 per cent sample or complete enumeration, is excluded from the discussion. Although sometimes employed [5], it is generally impractical and rarely undertaken for studies of large universes.

A distinguishing feature of probability samples is that each element of the universe has a known, nonzero probability of selection. Conversely, in nonprobability samples the probabilities of selection are unknown for some or all members, and some elements may have selection probabilities of zero occurring either as a deliberate choice by the investigator or through failure to define a universe clearly and to cover it completely. There is always some degree of error associated with estimates derived from sample data, and some sampling designs will yield more variable estimates than others. A real value in employing a probability design is that the magnitude of the sampling variation (error) can be calculated. From the sample, one can compute estimates for a definable universe.

Moreover, one can state what the chances are that a specified range above and below an estimate will encompass the population value. Such desirable characteristics are not shared by nonprobability samples.

Nonprobability Samples

In this monograph the term nonprobability is applied to samples which at some stage of sampling permit subjective choice of sampling units, the selection of some and the rejection of others being determined arbitrarily by the sampler. In some instances, the distinction between probability and nonprobability samples may be a matter of interpretation. For example, a rigorous probability selection of patients within a group of hospitals "willing to cooperate" is a proper probability selection from a universe defined as patients in the participating hospitals; the sample is not a probability selection of patients from a universe defined to include patients in nonparticipating hospitals. That is, the subjective selection of hospitals "willing to cooperate" should not be interpreted as yielding a probability sample of patients in the combined groups. While there is no intent to imply that nonprobability designs should never be used or that they always yield unreliable estimates, it must be emphasized that nonprobability samples provide no means within themselves to measure the precision of estimates, and in many situations there is no definable universe characterized by the estimates. Nonprobability samples may vary widely in complexity—from a subjective selection of a "handful" of patient records in one hospital to an objective selection of patient records in a group of hospitals judged by the investigator to reproduce the universe with respect to several important characteristics. In the latter instance, the researcher may come close to probability sampling but fail to achieve it because a probability of selection was not assigned to each institution in the universe.

Several terms are associated with nonprobability samples [6, 18, 19]. *Judgment sampling* involves some human element or judgment, presumed to be "good," in the selection procedure. *Chunk* sampling is applied to the selection of convenient sections of a universe; here, convenience more than good judgment may dictate the selection. *Purposive samples* are chosen to satisfy some predetermined purposes or criteria. If the purpose is to obtain certain numbers of subjects in assigned groups or classes (e.g., age, sex, or diagnosis), and the investigator is permitted some freedom of choice subject to the assigned restrictions, then the term *quota sampling* applies. An objective of each of these selection procedures is to choose samples "typical" or "representative" of some universe.

Chunk sampling of patient stays, as an illustration of nonprobability sampling, usually consists of taking a convenient batch of medical records but assumes an air of quasi-sophistication by specifying, for example, selection of all patients discharged during a "typical" week, or month, or from a "typical" nursing unit. The elements chosen by this particular method may or may not be "representative" of the population the researcher is interested in describing; the point is that no one knows. The choice of the "typical" population segment is dependent upon someone's judgment and defies attachment of any degree of certainty to the results. A chunk sampling counterpart for hospitals is "all hospitals of average size," or all hospitals in a "typical" region or area. A type of "representative" or quota sample, showing more sophistication, is that of matched pairs of patients sometimes used in studying two kinds of treatment. Under this plan, pairs of patients are chosen by controlling on certain characteristics—perhaps diagnosis, age, and sex. But rarely is any attempt made to determine the probabilities of selection within a group.

The widespread use of judgment samples in many research areas [29] resulted from a need for information developing faster than sampling techniques. In spite of recent advances in probability sampling methods, judgment samples continue to flourish at least in part because they are considered by some investigators to have advantages over probability samples with respect to cost and administrative convenience. Although the theory of simple random sampling is of long standing, applications of sampling techniques to practical problems are of more recent origin, having developed during the present century and at a pace more rapid than publication of accompanying theory or the training of sampling technicians. However, with current journal articles and several recently published books making modern probability sampling techniques generally available, the continued use of nonprobability samples is less justifiable.

Probability Samples

One aim of modern probability sampling methods is to provide maximum precision per dollar invested. A wide variety of sampling procedures enables the technician to design an efficient sample to meet the demands of a particular study. This variety of sampling techniques has a disadvantage in that nontechnicians may view probability procedures as too complex for easy understanding and hence to be avoided. The choice of an appropriate probability sampling design depends upon the research objectives, time, resources, and skill of the investigator. Some designs are inherently more efficient than others. It is important to note that in probability sampling the researcher can specify in advance just how much error he is willing to tolerate in the estimates and, with the help of a sampling statistician, choose a plan to ensure that the error falls within the tolerable limits. Another advantage of sampling, sometime overlooked, is that observations or measurements frequently can be made more accurately on a sample of cases than on the whole population. As an example, during the data collection phase of the study of the "Character and Effectiveness of Hospital Use," the two field teams obtained basic demographic and diagnostic information on 10,000 patients discharged during 1958 and abstracted in great detail the medical records of the 6,000 who had one of 18 diagnoses of special interest to the effectiveness study. If the entire population of cases in the 18 diagnoses had been included, the magnitude of the task would have increased a hundredfold. There was neither time nor money available for the constant supervision and painstaking verification processes associated with abstracting nearly a half-million medical records. Undetected clerical errors and failure to locate and transcribe records temporarily absent from the files can result in biases of greater magnitude than the errors of estimates derived from only a sample of cases.

Probability samples are of different types, some simple in concept and operation, others more complex. Although each may at some time be employed in sampling either hospitals or patients, no attempt will be made to discuss all sampling techniques or to give a "cookbook" solution to sampling problems. Here the objective is to describe or define and illustrate a few basic types of probability samples. The reader who entertains the idea of using some sampling device is directed to several excellent sources [2, 4, 6, 7, 18, 20] and is encouraged to seek expert assistance in choosing an efficient design for the job at hand.

SIMPLE RANDOM SAMPLING

In this design, every unit in the population is assured an equal and independent chance of selection. As an example, assume that a simple random sample of 300 admissions is to be chosen from 15,000 admissions to a 400-bed hospital during a particular year. The mechanics of case selection would be:

1. Number consecutively, from 1 to 15,000, each entry in the admission ledger, or list, for the specified year.

2. Using a table of random numbers [10], draw 300 different numbers in the range 1 through 15,000, ignoring duplicates of those that have already been drawn [18, pp. 116–118]. (This is known as "sampling without replacement." The departure from sampling with replacement after each selection is taken into account by a correction factor in the computations of standard errors of estimates [9, pp. 42–43].)

3. Select from the admission list the identification information for patients whose assigned numbers correspond with the chosen random numbers.

Now suppose the task is to select a sample of *persons* admitted to the hospital during the study period. It is possible that some individuals had multiple admissions during the year, so their names appear more than once on the admission list. One could go painstakingly through the list and eliminate all repetitions, but the magnitude of the task plus the possibility that two or more patients had the same name might prove discouraging. The deletion process would be facilitated in those hospitals using the unit record system, i.e., a unique, permanent number for each patient admitted.

But suppose that an admission listing is to be used. Assume also that a self-weighting sample (one in which sample elements have equal weight in analysis) is desired. Then the procedure would be:

1. Number each entry in the admission ledger as before.

2. Draw, say, 350 different random numbers (the exact multiple of the needed sample size will depend upon the estimated magnitude of repeated admissions to the particular hospital).

3. Select from the admission list the identification information for patients whose assigned numbers correspond with the chosen random numbers.

4. Retain a patient in the sample if and only if his first admission for the study period has been selected. This determination is made in two steps:
    a) If two or more hospital stays appear in the sample for the same patient, eliminate the later stay, keeping only the chronologically earlier one.
    b) From a master file or other source, determine if the particular sample stay for the patient was the *first during the study period*. If there was an earlier admission, eliminate the selected admission from the sample.

A sample of persons thus selected will be a self-weighting one for the time period of the study.

As can be seen, "simple" random sampling is something of a misnomer. The clerical work involved can, in some situations, be enormous. Furthermore, the investigator may want to insure that the selected cases are spread throughout the study period in order to estimate seasonal fluctuations—in bed occupancy or diagnostic distribution, for examples. Some sample designs make use of foreknown patient characteristics, achieving under favorable conditions a higher degree of precision than with simple random samples of the same size. The technique employed in such designs is stratification.

STRATIFIED SAMPLING

As the name implies, stratified sampling consists of dividing the patient population into homogeneous groups (strata) according to some
characteristic such as type of service (medical, surgical, OB-GYN, etc.),
nursing unit, or source of payment and selecting a separate sample *within*
each stratum. Each patient is placed in one and only one stratum before
sampling. If measurements are made on an adequate sample of each
stratum, separate estimates may be computed by stratum; the strata
estimates, when appropriately combined, form estimates for the total
population. The patient characteristic chosen for stratification purposes
should have a reasonably high correlation (usually a subjective evaluation determined by inspection or based on experience) with the variable
under investigation. An objective of stratification is to minimize differences within a stratum and to maximize differences among strata.

As an illustration, consider that the degree of patient satisfaction with
the nursing care in a particular hospital is to be determined. Abdellah and
Levine [1], in a recent study of the effect of nurse staffing on satisfactions with nursing care, found that patients reported fewer unfulfilled
needs in hospitals providing a higher number of hours of professional
nursing care per patient day, and that obstetrical patients reported approximately the same proportion of unfulfilled needs, regardless of how
much or what type of nursing care was provided. New, Nite, and Callahan
[24] also found that favorable patient opinions concerning the adequacy
of nursing care were positively related to a high number of nursing hours
available per patient. Furthermore, they found patients held more favorable opinions in those nursing units which had a higher ratio of RN's to
total staff, controlling on the total number of nursing hours available.
Selected findings from these two studies indicate that a useful variable
for stratification might be whether the patient was in the medical, surgical, or OB-GYN division of the hospital, or whether he was cared for in a
nursing unit with a "high," "medium," or "low" ratio of RN's to total
staff.

As Kish has pointed out [20, pp. 191–192], a stratified sampling technique has three principal advantages: (1) greater precision is obtained
for the sample estimates through the reduction of the variances of the
sample results for the total population; (2) it enables the investigator to
use different selection procedures within the various strata, if desired;
and (3) estimates of some stated precision can be constructed for each
subpopulation (stratum) separately, as well as estimates for the entire
population.

There are several types of stratified samples. The number of cases
selected within each stratum may be equal or unequal, proportionate or
disproportionate to the total population. Choice of an appropriate strati-

fied sampling plan must ultimately depend upon the objectives of the research and should take into account the variation of elements within each stratum with respect to the variable under investigation.

Using the example of patient satisfaction with nursing care, assume that after reviewing the literature on the subject, the results of a pilot study in the hospital have led to a decision to divide the hospitalized population into three strata—the medical, surgical, and OB-GYN divisions of the hospital. A *proportionate stratified random sample* of patients discharged from these divisions during a specified time period would involve selecting a separate sample from each stratum as outlined under the previous discussion of simple random sampling, using the same sampling fraction in each.

In Illustration A, distribution of the universe of patients in a hypothetical hospital is shown, with the number of discharges and the proportions of the total population in each stratum. Assuming a total sample size of 600 and a constant sampling fraction of 1/25, it is a simple matter to calculate the number of cases to be selected from each division. For patients discharged from the medical division, 280 random numbers are to be chosen within the range beginning with 1 and continuing through 7,000; 200 random numbers, 1 through 5,000, are required for patients discharged from the surgical division; and for patients discharged from the OB-GYN division, 120 numbers from 1 through 3,000 are to be selected. Under this plan the sample is self-weighting, meaning that each sample case in each division has the same probability of selection for the sample and the same weight in analysis.

For special study the investigator may want to have the same number of sample cases (200) from each division. This would be an example of a *disproportionate* stratified sample and would necessitate unequal weighting of the cases for a total population estimate. Illustration A gives the distribution of responses that might have been obtained in such a sample (column 8). The computation of the proportion of patients with favorable opinions in each stratum (column 9) merely involves dividing the number of patients holding these opinions by the total number of cases in the stratum. However, to arrive at an estimate of the proportion of *all* patients having favorable opinions, a weighted average of the strata proportions (column 9) is required—the respective weights being the proportion of discharges in a stratum (column 3). The calculation in footnote c of the illustration says that this weighted average is equal to the summation of the weighted proportions divided by the sum of the weights. (In this case, the denominator is 1.0. An alternate procedure yields the weighted strata proportions as well as their average by first calculating a weighted total for each stratum. See columns 10, 11 of the illustration.) Although the differential allocation of the sample may ap-

ILLUSTRATION A
Proportionate and disproportionate stratified sampling

Stratum	THE UNIVERSE		PROPORTIONATE SAMPLING		DISPROPORTIONATE SAMPLING						
							Patients with favorable opinions			
							The sample		Estimates for the universe	
	Number of discharges	Proportion of discharges[a]	Sample size	Sampling fraction	Sample size	Sampling fraction	Number	Proportion of stratum	Weighted total[b]	Proportion of total[c]
1	2	3	4	5	6	7	8	9	10	11
Total	15,000	1.000	600	1/25	600	...	319	...	8,255	.550
Medical	7,000	.467	280	1/25	200	1/35	150	.750	5,250	.350
Surgical	5,000	.333	200	1/25	200	1/25	47	.235	1,175	.078
OB-GYN	3,000	.200	120	1/25	200	1/15	122	.610	1,830	.122

[a] Used as weights when combining strata to form estimate for total population.

[b] The weighted total for each stratum is the number of favorable opinions inflated by the reciprocal of the sampling fraction; for example, 5,250 = 150 × 35.

[c] $.550 = \dfrac{(.467 \times .750) + (.333 \times .235) + (.200 \times .610)}{.467 + .333 + .200}$. Also, $.550 = \dfrac{8,255}{15,000}$.

pear to be an unnecessarily complex procedure, it is usually justified by cost considerations, the relative facility with which the information may be gathered in each stratum, and, most importantly, by the variation within each stratum.

The advantages of stratified sampling over simple random sampling are accompanied by a few disadvantages: (1) the practical difficulties inherent in choosing a simple random sample are still present since a simple random sample is selected in each stratum; (2) the investigator must have prior knowledge of the relationship between the variable of interest and those available for stratification; (3) furthermore, he must be able to assign each population element to a stratum on the basis of the stratification variable before sampling;[1] (4) unless there are large differences among the strata with respect to the variable under investigation, gains in precision by using stratified sampling rather than simple random sampling are slight (in fact, under certain conditions stratified sampling may result in less precision than would have been obtained with simple random sampling [18, p. 204; 2, p. 76]); and finally, (5) there is usually more than one variable under investigation in a particular research project. A stratified sample constructed to estimate one variable with increased precision may result in less precise estimates for other variables. For instance, if we were interested also in estimating the degree of patient satisfaction with prepaid health insurance plans, hospital division may not be a proper choice for stratification.

SYSTEMATIC SAMPLING

Simple random sampling and stratified simple random sampling both involve considerable clerical labor in the selection operation. In the hospital setting, selection of patients is frequently accomplished by working with a list or card file of admissions to or discharges from a particular institution. An alternative to numbering each patient in the population and then choosing random numbers to designate the sample is to take an interval, or systematic, sample. By this technique the sample is composed of every kth individual selected from a list or card file of patients after a random start equal to or less than k but greater than zero. An immediately apparent advantage is that usually only one random number must be chosen—the remaining cases being designated by successive additions of the interval k to the random start. The illustration of the selection of a sample of 300 hospital admissions from a universe of 15,000 used in the discussion of simple random sampling can be adapted to systematic selection. The investigator first computes the sampling interval

$$k = \frac{\text{total number of cases in the population}}{\text{number of cases needed in sample}} ;$$

---

[1] It is possible to use a technique of post-stratification not discussed here [18, p. 232].

he then chooses a random number greater than zero but not exceeding k. Counting along the list, the first selection is the individual denoted by the random number, and every kth individual thereafter is also designated for the sample. In the example, the sampling interval would be

$$k = \frac{N}{n} = \frac{15{,}000}{300} = 50 \; ,$$

so that one first chooses a random number in the range 1 through 50. Suppose 27 was chosen. The 27th case on the list would be the first sample selection; then merely adding 50 identifies the next sample case, and so on. The procedure is continued taking every 50th until the elements on the list are exhausted. The first several selections would be cases numbered 27, 77, 127, 177, 227, 277, 327, etc.

A population list to be sampled is ordered in *some* fashion: chronological, alphabetical, by nursing unit, by discharge, or the like. The ordering of patients on the list is extremely important in determining the nature of the sample selected. In some circumstances the ordering creates a systematic bias in the sample and the actual mechanics of selection should be altered. If the 15,000 admissions in the hypothetical patient population were thoroughly shuffled and then listed, a systematic sample would be equivalent to a simple random sample of the same size. If the admissions were in chronological order by time of admission, the results of systematic selection would approximate proportionate sampling of patients stratified by month of the year admitted.

In applying an interval to a list or file, one should be wary of a possible cyclic effect that tends to overselect one *type* of patient and underselect another type. For example, if a sample of admissions is selected from a list compiled daily of all patients admitted on that day, listed under the nursing unit to which they were assigned, and the ordering of nursing units kept constant throughout the year, then under these conditions it is possible that a disproportionate number of cases admitted to one nursing unit (say, pediatrics) would be selected, and the sample would be loaded with patients in younger age groups. If the possibility of cyclic fluctuation exists, systematic sampling either should be avoided or modified in some way to avoid possible bias. A common alteration is random selection *within* each interval. Frequently, this is accomplished by dividing the universe into groups corresponding to the size of the interval and choosing a different random number within each.

It is evident that the clerical work in systematic selection will increase in proportion to the length of a list or the number of file cards to be sampled. In fact, the systematic selection of every kth unit from a large population may become prohibitively time-consuming and expensive. A search for some means of reducing sampling costs led to the development of another sampling technique—that of cluster sampling.

CLUSTER SAMPLING

Cluster sampling is a term applied to a sampling procedure which selects population elements in groups or clusters. For example, instead of counting through all pages of a hospital admissions ledger to select a systematic sample of patients, one may select first a sample of ledger pages, then include all or some fraction of the patients listed on the sample pages. The patients selected from one page comprise one cluster, and the number of sample clusters would equal the number of sample pages.

Cluster sampling of card files may be effected by first choosing a sample of file drawers and subselecting cards within sample drawers. Here a sample cluster is composed of sample cards from one file drawer.

Properly designed cluster samples may prove to be more efficient than those selected by means of other methods which have been described. That is, under favorable conditions and for a specified degree of sampling variability, cluster sampling may yield the desired estimates at less cost than would be entailed with other sampling methods. Conditions favoring cluster sampling are: (1) the clusters can be easily and uniquely defined and identified; (2) once a sample element has been located, data collection costs are relatively low for additional, nearby elements; (3) the members of a cluster are sufficiently dissimilar to justify the inclusion of additional elements beyond the first. Frequently cluster samples require a larger sample size than would simple random sampling to produce estimates with specified sampling variability. Thus, for over-all costs to be lower, savings on sampling and data collection of cluster samples must be large enough to compensate for the costs of processing a larger sample and analyzing a more complex one.

Cluster sampling may succeed when other types of probability samples are virtually impossible to execute because of practical difficulties. Such a situation arises with a national, state, or even a metropolitan study of hospital care. The difficulties of compiling patient lists for purposes of simple random or systematic selections are insurmountable. However, by employing cluster sampling, the investigator may select a sample of hospitals and subselect patients within hospitals, the sample patients from each hospital comprising a cluster. Usually a list of hospitals can be compiled for a large area when the listing of patients cannot be accomplished.

There are special techniques for efficient sampling of large clusters of unequal size, such as hospitals which vary from a few beds to several thousand beds. Giving equal probability of selection to hospitals might seriously affect the precision of estimates. A preliminary step requires defining size and assigning a measure of size to each hospital. Size may be interpreted as number of beds, number of annual discharges, or average daily census, for examples. One technique, known as sampling with probability proportionate to size [18, p. 341], assigns to a hospital a probability of selection in proportion to its measure; sampling of patients within a hospital is then inversely proportional to the hospital measure of size. By this method hospitals with many beds (discharges, or patients) have greater chances of selection than hospitals with few beds. However, approximately equal numbers of patients would be selected from the sample hospitals. Thus, the objective to reduce variability in the ultimate cluster size is achieved.

A second technique relies on stratification to control variation in size of hospitals [18, p. 348]. By this method, several size classes are established and each hospital is assigned to one group. Within a group, the sampling of hospitals is with equal probability. Sampling among the large hospitals is at a high rate, while the selection rate declines as average size of hospital declines. The sampling of patients within hospitals follows a reverse pattern, being high in the small hospitals and low in the large ones. This technique was combined with controlled selection to choose the Michigan sample of hospitals and patients described in Chapter III.

CONTROLLED SELECTION

In the words of Goodman and Kish, controlled selection is defined to mean [16]

. . . any process of selection in which, while maintaining the assigned probability for each unit, the probabilities of selection for some or all preferred combinations of n out of N units are larger than in stratified random sampling (and correspondingly the probabilities of selection for at least some nonpreferred combinations are smaller than in stratified random sampling).

It is to be noted that while in stratified random sampling the probabilities of selection for certain combinations are increased, the possibilities of increasing the probabilities of selection for preferred combinations are by no means exhausted by this process. That is, with controlled selection it is in general possible to go very much further in increasing the probabilities of selection of preferred combinations of units than is done by stratified sampling alone. At the same time the probability of selection for vast numbers of other combinations is reduced, generally to zero. It is with the use of controls after the possibilities of stratification have been exhausted that controlled selection is concerned.

. . . .

Conceptually, the use of controls in selecting a sample may be viewed as an extension of the technique known as purposive selection (although perhaps involving more judgment). If, however, the estimates to be derived from the sample are to be unbiased, an additional step not ordinarily considered to be a part of purposive selection is required. In order that the sampling may be probability sampling, the sampler must select not just one but many purposive samples, until every unit in the universe is included in one or more samples. The number of samples in which each unit appears must be exactly proportionate to its assigned probability of selection.

After the complete set of purposive samples has been established, the random selection of one of them constitutes a probability sample. . . .

There is a frequently encountered misconception that probability sampling cannot be used for "small" samples, but a small number of sampling units can be chosen subjectively to reflect the variability of the universe. Little publicized and unknown to many investigators, controlled selection is a technique developed to increase the likelihood (over that of random sampling) of choosing a preferred, purposive combination of sampling units *while maintaining probability methods.* It may be regarded as a form of stratification which also controls the combinations of sampling units that may appear together in any sample. The selection procedure is particularly applicable to "large," first-stage sampling units (such as hospitals, schools, counties) when stratification by many variables is desired and the number of sample selections is relatively small. However, the technique may be used in singlestage sampling (or at any level of multistage sampling), when either more or fewer selections are to be made, and whenever only limited stratification is required.

The probability method resembles the judgment selection in that many purposive combinations of sampling units are formed but only one is chosen as the sample. A major distinction is this: in the subjective approach, many combinations may be examined and discarded, the determination of the sampling units being arbitrary; with the probability technique, purposive combinations are recorded and assigned probabilities of selection, the final choice being a *probability selection* from a set of combinations. In controlled selection, no unit is excluded with certainty, and the subjective determination relates to *stratification*—not to sample selection.

Essential conditions of controlled selection are: (1) each sampling unit must have an assigned, nonzero probability of selection; (2) the number of selections is determined prior to the controlled selection; (3) patterns (preferred combinations of sampling units) are formed and assigned a probability of selection subject to the restrictions of selection probabilities of individual units and the total number of selections; (4) pattern formation must continue until each unit has its proper probability of selection and the cumulative pattern probability equals exactly 1; (5) the selection of a single pattern is made at random (by choosing a random number) from a complete set of patterns with probabilities totaling 1 over the set.

Illustration B contains a simple example of a situation where all possible selection combinations, preferred and nonpreferred, can be listed. Then the example demonstrates that through the use of controlled selection the probability of choosing a preferred combination is increased from .5 to .9 while the probability of choosing a nonpreferred combination is reduced to 0.1. This is the essence of controlled selection: to increase the probability of selection for preferred combinations of sampling units and

ILLUSTRATION B

Controlled selection in a simple sampling situation

[Sampling plan: One hospital to be selected with equal probability from each group; preferably the selections will have different ownership codes]

1. Hospitals of a city, classified by size and ownership

Large hospitals			Small hospitals		
Hospital code	Ownership code	Probability of selection	Hospital code	Ownership code	Probability of selection
A	1	.25	a	1	.20
B	1	.25	b	1	.20
C	2	.25	c	2	.20
D	2	.25	d	2	.20
			e	2	.20
Total	. . .	1.00	. . .	. . .	1.00

2. All possible selection combinations of large and small hospitals if one hospital is selected at random from each stratum

1. A a	6. B a	11. C a *	16. D a *
2. A b	7. B b	12. C b *	17. D b *
3. A c *	8. B c *	13. C c	18. D c
4. A d *	9. B d *	14. C d	19. D d
5. A e *	10. B e *	15. C e	20. D e

* Preferred combinations of ownership codes.

Note: 1.   Each combination has equal probability of selection, .25 × .20 = .05, and the sum of the probabilities over 20 combinations = 1.00.
   2.   Each large hospital has selection probability 5 × .05 = .25.
   3.   Each small hospital has selection probability 4 × .05 = .20.
   4.   The probability of selecting a preferred combination is 10/20 = .5.

to reduce the probability of selection (preferably, but not necessarily, to zero) of nonpreferred combinations while maintaining a preassigned, non-zero probability of selection for each sampling unit.

The application of controlled selection to a more complex sampling problem is demonstrated in Chapter III.

FURTHER CONSIDERATIONS IN PROBABILITY SAMPLING

Sample selection is only one aspect of probability sampling which, if it is to fulfill an objective to provide maximum precision per unit of cost, must be concerned with many phases of research encompassed in the general term of sample design. This, in turn, is only part of the over-all project or study design.

ILLUSTRATION B—Continued

3. Controlled selection used to increase selection probabilities of preferred combinations from 0.5 to 0.9.

Pattern number	1	2	3	4	5	6	7	8
Pattern probability	.20	.20	.20	.20	.05	.05	.05	.05
Cumulative probability	.20	.40	.60	.80	.85	.90	.95	1.00
Combination of hospitals	A c *	B d *	C a *	D b *	A e *	B e *	C e	D e

Alternate set of patterns

Pattern number	1	2	3	4	5	6	7	8
Pattern probability	.05	.05	.05	.05	.20	.20	.20	.20
Cumulative probability	.05	.10	.15	.20	.40	.60	.80	1.00
Combination of hospitals	A c *	B c *	C c	D c	A d *	B e *	C b *	D a *

* Preferred combinations of ownership codes.

Note: 1. "Pattern" means any selection combination of one large and one small hospital.
2. A *preferred* pattern is one formed by hospitals of differing ownership.
3. Over one set of patterns, each large hospital appears in patterns with probabilities summing to .25, while a small hospital is included in patterns summing to .20. Therefore, each hospital has its proper probability of selection.
4. Since the probabilities of preferred patterns sum to .9, the probability of selecting a preferred combination is .9 and the probability of nonpreferred combinations has been reduced to .1.
5. The two sets of patterns do not exhaust all possible sets of combinations.
6. Each set need not have the same number of patterns; in this example the minimum number is 8 and the maximum 100. However, there cannot be 100 *different* patterns. The formation of a set of patterns is not complete until each hospital has its proper probability of selection and the cumulative probabilities over the set equal 1. These are simultaneous events. The ordering of patterns is arbitrary.
7. It is not wrong to include a nonpreferred pattern, e.g., C c. It *is* wasted effort to use controlled selection for nonpreferred combinations if they can be avoided.
8. When patterns are completed, the selection of a random number from 001 through 100 identifies a selected pattern. For example, random numbers 001 through 020 would select pattern 1 in the first set of patterns; random numbers 021 through 040 would select pattern 2, etc.
9. Refer to Chapter III for procedures generally followed in the formation of a set of patterns for an actual sampling situation.

Sample Design and Study Design

In addition to sample selection, sample design includes determination of the selection process to be used, calculation of sample size and sampling fractions, estimation procedures both for characteristics of the population and for sampling errors of such estimates. Study design goes beyond sample design to cover data collection and processing, control of non-sampling errors, analysis and presentation of findings.

Probability sampling has a salutary effect on the entire research design. Until he has thoughtfully considered research objectives and procedures, the investigator, who might otherwise postpone planning some phase of research, will find himself unable to answer questions raised by the sampling statistician who generally will inquire about the definition of the universe, the uses to be made of the data, availability of materials for sampling, types of estimates planned, desired precision of estimates, tabulation plans, and financial restrictions. Sometimes these inquiries lead to revision or even abandonment of a project because it is in some way un-realistic—for examples, objectives and concepts ill-defined, or too costly. More frequently, the free exchange of ideas and experiences results in improved research. Once there is agreement on objectives, estimation procedures, precision of estimates, and costs, sample size follows as a consequence of these decisions.

Sample Size

In advance of the selection of a probability sample, it is generally possible to estimate the size so as to be neither wastefully large nor disappointingly small. The investigator, however, is required to think through his research objectives, to decide what he wishes to estimate or measure and how precise the estimates need to be. Sample size is not so much a consequence of size of the universe as of precision of estimates. One does not necessarily take a "small" sample from a small universe, as one hospital, and a "large" sample from a large universe, which might be all hospitals of a state. Neither is there a magic number, such as 10 per cent, to yield an appropriate sample size under all conditions. Other factors remaining constant, for a specified degree of precision sample sizes do not differ widely even though the populations from which they are drawn vary considerably in size. Some of the principles involved can be illustrated with an example from simple random sampling.

Suppose a hospital administrator needs to know the proportion of patients with hospital bills *completely* paid by insurance carrier X. Ad-missions to the hospital number about 10,000 per year, and the only readily available source of information is individual financial ledgers. For reasons of speed and economy there is a decision to obtain the information from a sample of ledgers to be selected from the universe of 10,000 admis-sion ledgers during the most recent calendar year. What is an appropriate sample size?

Assuming that the hospital record system makes simple random sam-pling feasible, two quantities, in addition to the size of the universe, are essential to the calculation of sample size: an approximate value for the characteristic to be estimated and the acceptable standard error of the estimate. Either the administrator will supply his best "guess" of the proportion of patients having bills paid by carrier X, or a preliminary tally of a random selection of ledgers, perhaps a hundred, will yield a crude estimate of the proportion. Suppose the estimate is 20 per cent.

It is unlikely that the administrator has even a slight notion of what might be a reasonable value for the standard error of the estimated proportion of patients with hospital bills paid by insurance carrier X. Through questioning, however, a sampling technician may establish that research objectives would be satisfied if there were a reasonably good chance that the proportion obtained by examining all patient records would be within a range of two percentage points on either side of the estimate obtained by examining a sample of records. "Reasonably good chance" may be interpreted as "19 chances in 20," a probability statement associated with a range of about two standard errors on either side of a sample mean. It is as though the administrator requested a sample design such that if the estimated characteristic is 20 per cent, then the chances would be 19 in 20 that the range 18 per cent to 22 per cent enclosed the proportion based on all 10,000 records.[2] When the range above and below the mean is two per cent, and the corresponding probability statement is that associated with two standard errors, it follows that one standard error is to be regarded as one per cent. (If the administrator wants virtual certainty that the proportion based on all records lies between 18 and 22 per cent provided that the proportion to be estimated is about 20 per cent, then three standard errors should be regarded as two per cent and one standard error as 0.67 per cent. This would require an increase of about 100 per cent in sample size.)

Now the quantities necessary to estimate the sample size are assembled. From knowledge of sampling technique [2, pp. 53–55], the sampler calculates the sample size, making use of the approximation

$$n = \frac{NPQ}{N(S.E.)^2 + PQ} ,$$

where n is the approximate sample size,
        N is the number of records in the universe,
        P is the proportion to be estimated,
        Q is $1 - P$,
        $S.E.$ is the standard error associated with the sample estimate.

With the values N $= 10,000$
                  P $= .2$
                  Q $= .8$
                  $S.E. = .01,$

an approximate value of n is

$$n = \frac{(10,000)(.2)(.8)}{10,000(.0001) + (.2)(.8)} = 1,379 \text{ or about } 1,380.$$

Since $10,000/1,380 = 7.2$, the administrator may decide to use a 1 in 7 sample and avoid decimals in the sampling interval of 7.2. Thus the sam-

---

[2] See Chapter V, footnote 7.

ple size would be about 1,400, a number considerably less than 10,000.[3] If a simple random sample of 1,400 records yields an estimate of about 20 per cent for the characteristic under study, the standard error will be approximately .01. On the other hand, if the sample estimate is noticeably different from 20 per cent, the standard error will deviate from .01. However, the probability statement still holds that the chances are 19 in 20 that a range of two standard errors on either side of the sample estimate will enclose the proportion based on complete coverage of records. The chances are 1 in 20 that the latter proportion lies outside the range just defined.

The preceding illustration is unrealistic in several respects: the opportunity to use simple random sampling arises infrequently; research objectives usually include the study of many variables rather than only one; sample size is not to be determined independent of cost considerations. For illustrative purposes the use of simple random sampling is justified since the calculations of sample sizes for more complex designs are beyond the scope of this monograph. Furthermore, if there were many study variables, the calculations of sample size could be based on the most important one. Or the investigator may compute the sample sizes for several important items and choose subjectively among them if the variations in size are not large. With marked variability in sample sizes, the investigator is advised to seek the assistance of an expert [2, p. 57–58]. Although the introduction of cost factors as well as precision of estimates in the calculation of sample size does not alter the general principles illustrated, it does lead to considerations of optimum design—a major contribution of probability sampling.

---

[3] Notice that if the universe were extended to $N = 100,000$ (which might be the situation if all hospitals of an urban area were included) and all other conditions held constant, then

$$n = \frac{(100,000)(.2)(.8)}{100,000(.0001) + (.2)(.8)} = 1,575.$$

Similarly, $N = 1,000,000$, and $N = 10,000,000$ would result in approximate sample sizes of 1,597 and 1,600, respectively. These calculations are summarized below:

N	n	n/N
10,000	1,380	.14 or about 1/7
100,000	1,575	.016 or about 1/64
1,000,000	1,597	.0016 or about 1/626
10,000,000	1,600	.00016 or about 1/6250

It is evident that the sample size has approached and will remain at 1,600 even though N continues to increase and the sampling fraction, n/N, to decrease. This demonstration verifies an earlier statement that for a given sampling procedure, precision of estimates has a stronger influence on sample size than does size of universe, equal precision requiring approximately equal sample sizes.

The qualification "approximately equal" covers the range 1,380 to 1,600 in the illustration. Furthermore, if the calculations were extended to smaller values for the universe, there would be corresponding decreases in the sample size. A factor to be considered is the *ratio* of the sample to the universe; when the ratio is greater than 1/20, the values of n may be considerably less than those required when the universe is, for all practical purposes, infinite. The smaller ratios, however, are generally more common; hence, sample sizes often show only small changes with increases in size of universe.

Optimum Design

In many sampling situations, not just one but several probability designs could be constructed for the task at hand. An optimum design is one which will yield the required precision of estimates at minimum cost, or for a fixed cost will provide desired estimates with maximum possible precision. Once the types of estimates, the precision, and the cost relationships have been described, the sampling technician can compute and compare approximate costs and precisions of estimates for alternate sampling plans, then choose the most efficient—that is, the optimum. If several designs are equally efficient, the choice is arbitrary.

Because necessary data for the development of an optimum design are not easily assembled (sometimes pilot studies to collect data for design purposes are required), strict adherence to theory is practiced infrequently. Moreover, investment in planning and design should be somewhat in proportion to total research expenditures and the uses of research. A course of action for many research undertakings lies somewhere between the extremes of an expensive pilot study and little or no consideration of alternate sampling designs for the purpose of choosing an efficient one. For the more complex circumstances of cluster sampling in two or more stages, some general cost and precision functions have been developed to guide the investigator to sample allocations that are close to optimum [2, p. 225 ff.; 18, Chs. 6, 7, and 8]. When a continuing research operation is undertaken, or repeated use of a sample design contemplated, the researcher would do well to invest some funds in sample design development to meet the special research needs.

Nonsampling Errors

Some investigators hold the opinion, and properly so, that if probability sampling is to be more than an empty phrase, the execution of the design requires high standards of achievement in all nonsampling phases of research. While it is true that refined sampling techniques cannot compensate for deficiencies in other research operations (e.g., transcription and abstraction of medical records), it is unrealistic to expect flawless performance. However, the existence of nonsampling errors is not a justification for poor sampling techniques but an opportunity, through control measures, to raise the quality of nonsampling activities.

Chapter III

Selecting the Michigan Sample
of General Hospitals and Patients

In the preceding chapters, objectives of the Michigan *Study of Hospital and Medical Economics* were presented and some general types of probability sampling techniques discussed. In this chapter, the sample selection of general hospitals and discharges is described, illustrating the application of probability techniques to a practical research problem. Although the description is specific to the Michigan study, the controlled selection of hospitals and the sampling of hospital records have general applicability in the field of hospital and medical care. For this reason and because the reader may be encountering controlled selection procedures for the first time, the technique is displayed in detail to provide experience which the researcher may transfer to his own sampling situation.

THE GENERAL DESIGN

With respect to general hospitals for short-term care, defined as average stay under 30 days, there were two major research areas: studies of the population of patients admitted to or discharged from hospitals, and studies of hospitals as institutions. Although sampling procedures apply equally well to admissions or discharges, the latter has the advantage of including only patients who have completed their hospital stays.

Two independent samples of general hospitals might have been drawn, one for the studies of discharges and another for studies of institutions. But the selection and execution of two samples would have increased study costs while sacrificing the comprehensiveness of research achieved by conducting both types of studies in a basic core of institutions. That is, the findings of different studies on the same sample hospitals can be interwoven and interpretations of the data made accordingly.

To satisfy the aims of the discharge studies it was desirable that the design provide: (1) a self-weighting, cross-section sample of discharges; (2) estimates by several hospital size groups and for several geographic areas, as well as for the state; (3) relatively simple procedures whereby discharges could be subsampled or supplemented by diagnostic category as judged necessary; (4) appropriate representation of hospitals with respect to type (whether medical or osteopathic),[1] ownership, accreditation, and Blue Cross participation, in addition to size and geographic location listed under (2).

It was thought that studies of institutions would be concerned primarily with hospital size as a variable, with less interest in geographic distribution, and more emphasis on hospital characteristics by type and ownership. In addition, rates of occupancy and per diem costs were basic to one study. Therefore, to ensure that the sample of hospitals would be large enough within each domain of study, simple procedures for supplementation and subsampling of institutions were essential.

The primary consideration of the research, both for studies of discharges and of institutions, was to provide valid estimates on which decisions affecting the medical economics of the state might be based. Clearly, probability sampling was dictated. Just as clearly, the situation demanded a controlled selection procedure to construct a master sample which would reflect the complex universe of hospitals and satisfy the specifications of research design.

Definitions and Preparatory Work

The Universe

Since the universe of hospitals is changing constantly, it was defined and listed for a specific study period—the most recent calendar year, 1958. A full year was a minimum requirement in order that the study reflect variations in hospital and medical care by days, weeks, months and seasons. The calendar year 1958 was selected both to coincide with the study periods of other phases of the *Study of Hospital and Medical Economics* and to circumvent problems related to the availability of patient data. The choice of the study period is extremely important when detailed medical or financial information for individual patients is needed to satisfy the objectives of the research. A study period that is too recent, in the sense of being too near the period of investigation, will encounter a sizeable proportion of incomplete medical records, outstanding financial accounts, and a multitude of problems related to record accessibility. A study period that is too distant from the research date may have to contend with "permanently" filed or misplaced medical records and destroyed financial ledger cards.

A list of Michigan hospitals, medical and osteopathic, devoted wholly or in part to short-term care was compiled and information obtained on important characteristics of each hospital. Among the characteristics were: number of beds, both total and general; type of hospital; owner-

---

[1] In this monograph, the terms "medical" and "osteopathic" are used as a matter of convenience and not because of any clear-cut distinction between the two types of general hospitals.

ship; Blue Cross participation; accreditation; and city and county of location.

In 1959 there was no one source from which a complete listing of the universe could be obtained. Lists and detailed information were provided by the American Hospital Association [17], the Office of Hospital Survey and Construction (Hill-Burton), Michigan Hospital Association, Michigan Osteopathic Hospital Association, Greater Detroit Area Hospital Council, Michigan Department of Health, and Michigan Hospital Service (Blue Cross). When essential information was not available elsewhere, it was obtained directly from the hospital.

Hospital Size

With some precedent both in the literature and in practice for expressing size in terms of beds, five size groups were thought to be meaningful and to have general applicability:

1. 500 or more beds;
2. 250–499 beds;
3. 100–249 beds;
4. 50–99 beds;
5. less than 50 beds.

Class boundaries, arbitrarily chosen, are not to be thought of as fine lines of distinction among hospitals but more as a convenience for purposes of sampling and analysis. One bed more or less does not change the character of a hospital even though the classification changes.

To classify a hospital by size, the number of beds it had set up, permanently available, for use during the entire study period was considered acceptable for the requirements of both analysis and sampling. If a hospital had separate facilities for special types of services (mental, T.B., custodial care), then only beds used for general, short-term care were included for the sample of discharges, inasmuch as discharges from these special facilities were excluded from the study universe.[2] Using total rather than general beds to determine size may, when they differ appreciably, cause the misclassification of a hospital and result in increased sampling variability.[3]

Geographic Districts

Six geographic districts, outlined in Figure 1, were defined after carefully considering patterns of hospital care throughout the state; differences in hospital utilization, costs and charges for services; and segments of the population subscribing to the Blue Cross program, or insured by

---

[2] These special facilities were added to the universe of "special" hospitals, and sampled separately. That sample will not be discussed in this monograph [11].

[3] Occasionally, it may be desirable to use total beds as a measure to classify a hospital for the study of institutions, and general beds as the measure for the discharge study. In this situation some technical assistance is advisable to resolve sampling complications.

commercial carriers. The districts are a function of the geography and general economy of the state as well as of hospital and medical economy. The upper peninsula is geographically isolated; the upper half of the lower peninsula is economically distinct. The remainder of the state has four divisions: the Detroit, and the Flint-Bay City-Saginaw areas to the east; the Grand Rapids-Muskegon area in the central and west; and the Lansing-Battle Creek-Kalamazoo area in the southwest.

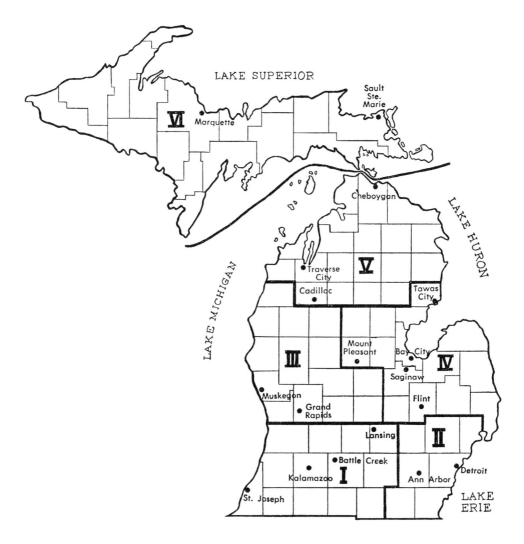

FIGURE 1. Division of the State of Michigan into Six Geographic Districts for the Study of Hospital and Medical Economics

SAMPLE SIZE AND OVER-ALL SAMPLING FRACTION

The sample size was determined to meet the objectives of the study of the "Character and Effectiveness of Hospital Use." Desired estimates for each of 35 diagnostic categories were:

1. average length of stay
2. average total hospital bill
3. distribution by primary source of payment of hospital bill
4. distribution by age of patient

Furthermore, for each of 18 diagnostic categories the effectiveness of hospital use was to be evaluated and the proportions of appropriate stays, overstays, and understays estimated; in addition, estimates of consumption of laboratory procedures and diagnostic x-ray were needed (both expressed as average number of units). A sample size of about 200 cases per diagnosis was desired for the 18 categories, in view of the analysis which was to include physician interviews for all inappropriate stays and for a subsample of appropriate stays.

Although sampling theory provides techniques to estimate sample size to produce maximum precision per dollar of cost within administrative restrictions, the sample size for this study was determined as that which would satisfy size requirements for the 18 diagnostic categories, within administrative restrictions but without specifying the precision of estimates. There were several reasons for this approach to sample size: demands on the study were numerous; approximate sampling errors of major study variables were unknown; cost data were not available; and the limitations on time did not permit a pilot study to collect data for sample design.

However, it was known that important estimates would be in the form of ratios (means, proportions) which, generally, would be less affected by variability among hospitals than estimates of aggregates might be. Furthermore, for the 18 diagnostic categories, per cent distributions of admissions by bed size groups were available from 22 PAS member hospitals in Michigan. These data permitted realistic assumptions about the per cent distributions of the 18 diagnoses in the universe of Michigan hospitals. Another essential preliminary figure was the approximate total number of discharges from all general hospitals in the state during 1958, estimated to be around 1,250,000.

To achieve a desired sample size of from 200 to 400 discharges per diagnostic category for a group comprising only one per cent of all discharges implied a sampling fraction ranging from around 1/60 to 1/30 and a total sample of 20,000 to 40,000 discharges. Since a sample of that magnitude was judged beyond the resources allocated for research, a sampling fraction around the midrange was selected as a compromise, with the idea that small groups could be supplemented by special techniques and large ones subsampled to keep the total sample around 10,000 discharges, thus saving the cost of collecting and processing data for an additional 15,000 or more cases that would be included if a constant sampling fraction were used. The over-all sampling fraction of 1/48 was chosen in preference to others of approximately that value because it has many factors, permitting separation into two components—a sampling fraction for hospitals, and one for discharges within hospitals.

CONTROLLED SELECTION OF HOSPITALS

Having clarified research objectives, definitions, and concepts, and after developing an over-all sampling fraction for the discharge studies, it was necessary to make an approximate determination of the number of sample hospitals that would be administratively feasible before the controlled selection of hospitals could progress beyond early stages. By estimating the number of man-hours required to complete the sampling and abstraction of records in one hospital, then comparing the estimates with figures on available funds, personnel, and time, it was determined that a maximum of about 50 hospitals would be practicable.

Stratification

Since separate estimates were desired by hospital size group and by geographic district, stratification by these two variables was essential. Geographic stratification was extended in district II to three substrata to ensure an appropriate probability selection from each: the city of Detroit, the remainder of the Standard Metropolitan Area, and the remainder of the district. Primarily because in 1958 the Joint Commission on Accreditation did not accredit any medical hospital with less than 25 beds, the group of hospitals with less than 50 beds was divided into those with 25 through 49 beds, and those with less than 25 beds; the latter was designated group 6. The type of general hospital was considered next in importance (after size and geography) as a stratification variable.

With this three-way stratification (six size groups, eight geographic areas, and two hospital types), there were 96 potential substrata which did not yet take into consideration the hospital characteristics of number of admissions, ownership, Blue Cross participation, accreditation, and county of location. To determine if controls should be imposed on these variables in the primary stage of selection, the characteristics of each hospital were posted on a file card and cards sorted into substrata defined by the three-way stratification. Cards within each substratum were examined to ascertain the degree of homogeneity of hospital characteristics. In some substrata all hospitals were accredited and Blue Cross-participating. The examination also revealed that: in all substrata a high proportion of hospitals were Blue Cross-participating; most of the non-

TABLE 1—Distribution of general medical and osteopathic hospitals, and number of beds, by geographic district and size group, State of Michigan, 1958

ITEM	TYPE OF HOSPITAL	STATE TOTAL		GROUP 1 (500 or more beds)		ALL OTHER GROUPS		GROUP 2 (250–499 beds)	
		Hosps.	Beds	Hosps.	Beds	Hosps.	Beds	Hosps.	Beds
STATE	Total	235	26,892	8	5,602	227	21,290	19	6,276
	Medical	200	24,717	8	5,602	192	19,115	18	5,881
	Osteopathic	35	2,175	0	0	35	2,175	1	395
DIST. I	Total	37	3,446	0	0	37	3,446	3	874
	Medical	32	3,241	0	0	32	3,241	3	874
	Osteopathic	5	205	0	0	5	205	0	0
DIST. II	Total	91	14,433	7	4,935	84	9,498	9	3,198
	Medical	77	13,144	7	4,935	70	8,209	8	2,803
	Osteopathic	14	1,289	0	0	14	1,289	1	395
DIST. III	Total	31	2,826	0	0	31	2,826	4	1,333
	Medical	23	2,483	0	0	23	2,483	4	1,333
	Osteopathic	8	343	0	0	8	343	0	0
DIST. IV	Total	38	3,841	1	667	37	3,174	3	871
	Medical	31	3,534	1	667	30	2,867	3	871
	Osteopathic	7	307	0	0	7	307	0	0
DIST. V	Total	16	939	0	0	16	939	0	0
	Medical	15	908	0	0	15	908	0	0
	Osteopathic	1	31	0	0	1	31	0	0
DIST. VI	Total	22	1,407	0	0	22	1,407	0	0
	Medical	22	1,407	0	0	22	1,407	0	0
	Osteopathic	0	0	0	0	0	0	0	0
Distrib. of beds (%)	Total	...	100.0	...	20.8	...	79.2	...	23.3
Avg. no. beds per hosp.	Total	...	114	...	700	...	94	...	330

accredited institutions were among the smaller size groups; with respect to hospital control, nonfederal governmental ownership was scattered among size groups, while church-operated or church-related institutions were generally among the larger hospitals, and proprietary ownership was associated more frequently with small hospitals; and number of admissions varied considerably within a substratum.

It appeared that gains resulting from increased controls (for example, three ownership classes) in the first stage of selection would be more than offset by the additional clerical work. Therefore, it seemed desirable to restrict primary controls to size, geography, and hospital type, deferring to a secondary selection stage the controls by ownership, accreditation, number of admissions, and Blue Cross participation.

The universe of general medical and osteopathic hospitals is displayed in Table 1, by six size groups and six geographic districts. (The substratification of district II is omitted but appears in later tables.) Table 1 also includes per cent distributions of beds, by size groups and geographic areas, and, for each size group, the average number of beds per hospital.

TABLE 1—(Continued)

ITEM	TYPE OF HOSPITAL	GROUP 3 (100–249 beds)		GROUP 4 (50–99 beds)		GROUP 5 (25–49 beds)		GROUP 6 (less than 25 beds)		DISTRIB. OF BEDS
		Hosps.	Beds	Hosps.	Beds	Hosps.	Beds	Hosps.	Beds	(%)
STATE	Total	55	8,361	57	3,947	56	2,047	40	659	100.0
	Medical	50	7,767	48	3,310	44	1,602	32	555	91.9
	Osteopathic	5	594	9	637	12	445	8	104	8.1
DIST. I	Total	9	1,368	13	856	7	263	5	85	12.8
	Medical	9	1,368	11	740	5	186	4	73	...
	Osteopathic	0	0	2	116	2	77	1	12	...
DIST. II	Total	26	3,997	21	1,509	17	608	11	186	53.7
	Medical	22	3,515	18	1,263	13	478	9	150	...
	Osteopathic	4	482	3	246	4	130	2	36	...
DIST. III	Total	3	409	11	741	8	273	5	70	10.5
	Medical	2	297	9	620	6	194	2	39	...
	Osteopathic	1	112	2	121	2	79	3	31	...
DIST. IV	Total	8	1,345	5	365	11	427	10	166	14.3
	Medical	8	1,345	3	211	8	299	8	141	...
	Osteopathic	0	0	2	154	3	128	2	25	...
DIST. V	Total	3	453	3	190	7	263	3	33	3.5
	Medical	3	453	3	190	6	232	3	33	...
	Osteopathic	0	0	0	0	1	31	0	0	...
DIST. VI	Total	6	789	4	286	6	213	6	119	5.2
	Medical	6	789	4	286	6	213	6	119	...
	Osteopathic	0	0	0	0	0	0	0	0	...
Distrib. of beds (%)	Total	...	31.1	...	14.7	...	7.6	...	2.5	...
Avg. no. beds	Total	...	152	...	69	...	37	...	16	...

These percentages and means were utilized when determining sampling fractions for the several size groups.

Sampling Fractions for Hospitals and Discharges

As stated earlier, the intent was to achieve a self-weighting, 1/48 sample of discharges by first sampling hospitals and then selecting discharges within the sample hospitals. Consistent with sampling theory [18, Ch. 8], research objectives, and administrative restrictions, for each hospital size group two sampling fractions were determined, one for each stage of sampling, with product 1/48.

When primary sampling units vary greatly in size, as do hospitals, it is efficient to equalize the number of patients selected from sample hospitals. This can be done by sampling large hospitals at high rates and small hospitals at low ones, then reversing the relationship of selection rates within hospitals to sample discharges at low rates in large hospitals and at high rates in small ones. In Table 1, it can be seen that from the largest to the smallest group the average number of beds per hospital roughly approximated a geometric series that progressed by a factor of about one-half. This suggested first-stage sampling fractions equal or proportional to 1, 1/2, 1/4, 1/8, and so on. Size group 1 contained the large teaching hospitals, those with research programs, specialized treatment centers, and with a large proportion of specialists on the medical staff; each of these institutions was considered unique and the research staff wished to include them with certainty. The pattern thus established for other size groups, following the preceding sequence, would have resulted in the selection of 43 or 44 hospitals, a number well within administrative restrictions. However, to increase the number of hospitals in the three small groups, permitting separate estimates for group 4 and for groups 5 and 6 in combination, and also to avoid a second-stage sampling fraction of 2/3 for group 6, the last three sampling fractions were changed to 1/6, 1/12, and 1/24, respectively.

Second-stage sampling fractions followed immediately, once first-stage fractions were determined; both are summarized with the expected hospital sample size, which was computed by applying a hospital sampling fraction to the appropriate number of hospitals in the universe:

Size group	Definition of size	Sampling fractions		Expected no. of sample hospitals
		For hospitals	For discharges	
1	500 or more beds	1:1	1:48	8.00
2	250–499 beds	1:2	1:24	9.50
3	100–249 beds	1:4	1:12	13.75
4	50–99 beds	1:6	1:8	9.50
5	25–49 beds	1:12	1:4	4.67
6	Less than 25 beds	1:24	1:2	1.67
	All size groups	. . .	1:48	47.09

In the controlled selection of hospitals, size group 1 was excluded inasmuch as the selection was completed with the inclusion of the eight institutions.

Determining the Number and Location of Selections To Be Made

The objective of controlled selection is to reduce the sampling variability of estimates obtained at a given cost. Since it enables the sampler to select a probability sample in accord with the universe as a whole with respect to as many hospital characteristics as the researcher considers important or desirable, it is particularly significant for a small sample of 39 or 40 hospitals. The method employed to carry out the selection procedure, described in detail with illustrations from the Michigan sample, is to be regarded as only one of several alternatives. Generally, each sample presents individual problems, and technicians prefer to develop their own system of record keeping. Specific operations to be discussed are: computing the expected sample size; determining selections to be decided by controlled techniques; preparation of worksheet and formation of selection patterns; maintaining control records; and choosing one pattern from the completed set.

COMPUTING THE EXPECTED SAMPLE SIZE

Having determined sampling fractions for hospital size groups, the next step was to compute the number of sample hospitals expected from each substratum of the universe to be sampled—that is, the 227 hospitals with less than 500 beds. Table 2 presents the distribution of hospitals by geographic district and type of hospital for the state and for size groups 2 through 6. The expected sample sizes were computed for substrata, then added by rows and columns to produce the marginal totals.

Within a size group the expected number of selections was determined by multiplying the number in the universe by the sampling fraction for the group. For example, the distribution of the 19 hospitals in group 2 (250–499 beds) throughout the first four districts is 3, 9, 4, 3. Since the sampling fraction is 1/2, the expected sample sizes are 1.5, 4.5, 2, and 1.5, or a total of 9.5 for the size group. Table 2 shows the allocations to medical and osteopathic hospitals as well as the totals by district. Since a hospital is regarded as a unit, the actual sample size would be either 9 or 10 hospitals. Continuing in this manner with the appropriate sampling fractions, the expected number of hospitals was computed for each cell of the table.

For the record, it is convenient to include in Table 2 the actual numbers of selections resulting from the controlled selection procedure, although in practice the sample selections are achieved not with such directness but only after considerable labor. The observant reader will notice that the selection of eight medical hospitals rather than the expected nine in the state total of group 2 is a flaw in an otherwise "perfect" set of selections—perfect in the sense that the actual number of selections for each of the other cells is within a fraction of the expected number. A different control on rounding errors in the selection process resulted in underselection of one medical hospital in group 2, but for all groups combined the number of selections was within expectation. The procedure described in the sections which follow eliminates this particular source of variability.

SELECTIONS TO BE DETERMINED BY CONTROLLED TECHNIQUES

In one sense, each of the 39 or 40 selections is to be determined by controlled techniques, but in the initial stage the controls serve to round the fractions in the sample expectations. That is, since we do not choose to select a fraction of a hospital, the controlled selection determines which fractional expectations are to be converted to 1's and which to 0's. Again

TABLE 2—Distribution of the universe,[a] the expected sample size and the actual number of selections, by geographic district, size group, and type of general hospital; State of Michigan, 1958

ITEM	TYPE OF HOSPITAL	TOTAL			GROUP 2 (250–499 beds)			GROUP 3 (100–249 beds)		
			Sample			Sample			Sample	
		Univ.	Exp.	Actual	Univ.	Exp.	Actual	Univ.	Exp.	Actual
STATE	Total	227	39.09	39	19	9.5	9	55	13.75	14
	Medical	192	34.51	34	18	9.0	8	50	12.50	13
	Osteopathic	35	4.58	5	1	.5	1	5	1.25	1
DIST. I	Total	37	6.71	7	3	1.5	1	9	2.25	3
	Medical	32	6.17	6	3	1.5	1	9	2.25	3
	Osteopathic	5	.54	1	0	.0	0	0	.00	0
DIST. II	Total	84	16.38	16	9	4.5	5	26	6.50	6
	Medical	70	13.96	14	8	4.0	4	22	5.50	5
	Osteopathic	14	2.41	2	1	.5	1	4	1.00	1
	Detroit city	40	8.62	9	5	2.5	3	14	3.50	3
	Medical	33	7.21	8	4	2.0	2	12	3.00	3
	Osteopathic	7	1.42	1	1	.5	1	2	.50	0
	Remainder of SMA[b]	32	5.75	5	3	1.5	1	10	2.50	3
	Medical	26	4.92	4	3	1.5	1	8	2.00	2
	Osteopathic	6	.83	1	0	.0	0	2	.50	1
	Remainder of District	12	2.00	2	1	.5	1	2	.50	0
	Medical	11	1.84	2	1	.5	1	2	.50	0
	Osteopathic	1	.17	0	0	.0	0	0	.00	0
DIST. III	Total	31	5.46	6	4	2.0	2	3	.75	1
	Medical	23	4.58	5	4	2.0	2	2	.50	1
	Osteopathic	8	.88	1	0	.0	0	1	.25	0
DIST. IV	Total	37	5.67	6	3	1.5	1	8	2.00	2
	Medical	30	5.00	5	3	1.5	1	8	2.00	2
	Osteopathic	7	.66	1	0	.0	0	0	.00	0
DIST. V	Total	16	1.96	2	0	.0	0	3	.75	1
	Medical	15	1.88	2	0	.0	0	3	.75	1
	Osteopathic	1	.08	0	0	.0	0	0	.00	0
DIST. VI	Total	22	2.92	2	0	.0	0	6	1.50	1
	Medical	22	2.92	2	0	.0	0	6	1.50	1
	Osteopathic	0	.00	0	0	.0	0	0	.00	0
Sampling fraction		...	...	...		1:2		...	1:4	

[a] Hospitals which are to be included with certainty have been excluded from the universe to be sampled.
[b] Wayne, Oakland and Macomb counties comprise the Detroit Standard Metropolitan Area (SMA).

looking at group 2 in Table 2 as an illustration, the expectation from district I is 1.5 medical hospitals. It is certain that at least one medical hospital is to be chosen. The uncertainty relates only to the fraction .5. Examining each cell of the table in this light leads to the realization that clerical labor can be reduced substantially if certainty selections are recognized and removed from the first phase of the controlled selection procedure, which need be concerned only with the allocation of noncertainty selections—that is, those whose locations are in doubt.

TABLE 2—(Continued)

Item	Type of Hospital	Group 4 (50 to 99 beds) Univ.	Sample Exp.	Sample Actual	Group 5 (25 to 49 beds) Univ.	Sample Exp.	Sample Actual	Group 6 (less than 25 beds) Univ.	Sample Exp.	Sample Actual
STATE	Total	57	9.50	10	56	4.67	5	40	1.67	1
	Medical	48	8.00	8	44	3.67	4	32	1.34	1
	Osteopathic	9	1.50	2	12	1.00	1	8	.33	0
DIST. I	Total	13	2.17	3	7	.58	0	5	.21	0
	Medical	11	1.83	2	5	.42	0	4	.17	0
	Osteopathic	2	.33	1	2	.17	0	1	.04	0
DIST. II	Total	21	3.50	3	17	1.42	2	11	.46	0
	Medical	18	3.00	3	13	1.08	2	9	.38	0
	Osteopathic	3	.50	0	4	.33	0	2	.08	0
	Detroit city	11	1.83	2	9	.75	1	1	.04	0
	Medical	10	1.67	2	6	.50	1	1	.04	0
	Osteopathic	1	.17	0	3	.25	0	0	.00	0
	Remainder of SMA[b]	5	.83	0	8	.67	1	6	.25	0
	Medical	4	.67	0	7	.58	1	4	.17	0
	Osteopathic	1	.17	0	1	.08	0	2	.08	0
	Remainder of District	5	.83	1	0	.00	0	4	.17	0
	Medical	4	.67	1	0	.00	0	4	.17	0
	Osteopathic	1	.17	0	0	.00	0	0	.00	0
DIST. III	Total	11	1.83	2	8	.67	1	5	.21	0
	Medical	9	1.50	2	6	.50	0	2	.08	0
	Osteopathic	2	.33	0	2	.17	1	3	.13	0
DIST. IV	Total	5	.83	1	11	.92	1	10	.42	1
	Medical	3	.50	0	8	.67	1	8	.33	1
	Osteopathic	2	.33	1	3	.25	0	2	.08	0
DIST. V	Total	3	.50	0	7	.58	1	3	.13	0
	Medical	3	.50	0	6	.50	1	3	.13	0
	Osteopathic	0	.00	0	1	.08	0	0	.00	0
DIST. VI	Total	4	.67	1	6	.50	0	6	.25	0
	Medical	4	.67	1	6	.50	0	6	.25	0
	Osteopathic	0	.00	0	0	.00	0	0	.00	0
Sampling fraction		...	1:6		...	1:12		...	1:24	

The illustration is carried forward to Table 3 where allocation of the total expected sample to certainty and noncertainty selections is shown. The subgroups from which 25 of the selections will come are already known. Controlled selection is needed to determine if the number of additional selections is to be 14 or 15, and from what district and size group each should come.

For illustrative purposes, computations in Table 3 were rounded to two decimals and adjusted to add to marginal totals; in an actual situation more precision in expected numbers may be desirable.

TABLE 3—Distribution of the expected sample of hospitals by certainty and noncertainty cells, State of Michigan

[Note: Numerical differences between Tables 2 and 3 are rounding errors. Figures in Table 3 have been forced to marginal totals by size group and type for each district and for the state]

Item	Type of Hospital	Total			Group 2			Group 3			Group 4			Group 5			Group 6		
		T[a]	C[a]	NC[a]	T	C	NC	T	C	NC	T	C	NC	T	C	NC	T	C	NC
1	2	3	4	5	3	4	5	3	4	5	3	4	5	3	4	5	3	4	5
State	Total	39.09	25.00	14.09	9.50	8.00	1.50	13.75	11.00	2.75	9.50	5.00	4.50	4.67	1.00	3.67	1.67	.00	1.67
	Medical	34.51	24.00	10.51	9.00	8.00	1.00	12.50	10.00	2.50	8.00	5.00	3.00	3.67	1.00	2.67	1.34	.00	1.34
	Osteopathic	4.58	1.00	3.58	.50	.00	.50	1.25	1.00	.25	1.50	.00	1.50	1.00	.00	1.00	.33	.00	.33
Dist. I	Total	6.72	4.00	2.72	1.50	1.00	.50	2.25	2.00	.25	2.17	1.00	1.17	.59	.00	.59	.21	.00	.21
	Medical	6.18	4.00	2.18	1.50	1.00	.50	2.25	2.00	.25	1.84	1.00	.84	.42	.00	.42	.17	.00	.17
	Osteopathic	.54	.00	.54	.00	.00	.00	.00	.00	.00	.33	.00	.33	.17	.00	.17	.04	.00	.04
Dist. II[b]	Total	16.37	14.00	2.37	4.50	4.00	.50	6.50	6.00	.50	3.50	3.00	.50	1.41	1.00	.41	.46	.00	.46
	Medical	13.96	13.00	.96	4.00	4.00	.00	5.50	5.00	.50	3.00	3.00	.00	1.08	1.00	.08	.38	.00	.38
	Osteopathic	2.41	1.00	1.41	.50	.00	.50	1.00	1.00	.00	.50	.00	.50	.33	.00	.33	.08	.00	.08
Dist. III	Total	5.46	3.00	2.46	2.00	2.00	.00	.75	.00	.75	1.83	1.00	.83	.67	.00	.67	.21	.00	.21
	Medical	4.58	3.00	1.58	2.00	2.00	.00	.50	.00	.50	1.50	1.00	.50	.50	.00	.50	.08	.00	.08
	Osteopathic	.88	.00	.88	.00	.00	.00	.25	.00	.25	.33	.00	.33	.17	.00	.17	.13	.00	.13
Dist. IV	Total	5.67	3.00	2.67	1.50	1.00	.50	2.00	2.00	.00	.84	.00	.84	.92	.00	.92	.41	.00	.41
	Medical	5.00	3.00	2.00	1.50	1.00	.50	2.00	2.00	.00	.50	.00	.50	.67	.00	.67	.33	.00	.33
	Osteopathic	.67	.00	.67	.00	.00	.00	.00	.00	.00	.34	.00	.34	.25	.00	.25	.08	.00	.08
Dist. V	Total	1.96	.00	1.96	.00	.00	.00	.75	.00	.75	.50	.00	.50	.58	.00	.58	.13	.00	.13
	Medical	1.88	.00	1.88	.00	.00	.00	.75	.00	.75	.50	.00	.50	.50	.00	.50	.13	.00	.13
	Osteopathic	.08	.00	.08	.00	.00	.00	.00	.00	.00	.00	.00	.00	.08	.00	.08	.00	.00	.00
Dist. VI	Total	2.91	1.00	1.91	.00	.00	.00	1.50	1.00	.50	.66	.00	.66	.50	.00	.50	.25	.00	.25
	Medical	2.91	1.00	1.91	.00	.00	.00	1.50	1.00	.50	.66	.00	.66	.50	.00	.50	.25	.00	.25
	Osteopathic	.00	.00	.00	.00	.00	.00	.00	.00	.00	.00	.00	.00	.00	.00	.00	.00	.00	.00

[a] The letters T, C and NC are to be interpreted as Total, Certainty and Noncertainty.

[b] District II included 7 counties in southeastern Michigan. For the controlled selection the district was divided into 3 parts: (1) Detroit city; (2) Remainder of Wayne, Oakland and Macomb Counties; (3) Remainder of district II (see Table 2). This had the effect of decreasing the number of certainty cells from 14 to 9, while the noncertainty increased to 7.37.

PREPARATION OF WORKSHEET AND FORMATION
OF SELECTION PATTERNS

Operationally, controlled selection consists in forming a complete set of purposive samples or patterns, each meeting the restrictions of the expected sample sizes for the substrata. The number of patterns cannot be specified in advance—there is no unique set—but the probability of selection must be known for each pattern and the probabilities over the set must add to 1.

Accurate records are imperative to the success of controlled selection. The worksheet presented and discussed in Illustration C is suggested as one way to record patterns and their selection probabilities. The display is designed to be self-explanatory.

When the expected sample sizes have been computed to two decimals, the minimum probability associated with a pattern is .01; the maximum value will vary with the specific pattern but must not exceed the minimum probability for subgroups included in the pattern, since the probability for the pattern also applies to each element in it. For example, the probability assigned to pattern 1 in Illustration C may vary from .01 to .17, the minimum probability of selection for subgroups comprising the pattern (see entries in column 3). Although the decision to use .05 is arbitrary, it results from experience which demonstrates that many patterns with small probabilities usually are more satisfactory than a few patterns with larger probabilities.

There are *minimum* requirements that each pattern should meet in the present example; these are the noncertainty selections appearing in Table 3 (column 5):

a) Reading across the first line of the table, there must be at least 14 selections in total; one from group 2, two from group 3, four from group 4, three from 5, and one from 6. The controlled selection appropriately distributes the remaining three selections among the size groups.

b) It is evident from line 2 that at least 10 medical hospitals are to be selected; one from group 2, two from group 3, three from group 4, two from 5, and one from 6; the location of the remaining selection is determined by the controlled operation.

c) At least three osteopathic hospitals are to be chosen: one from group 4, one from 5, one to be determined by the selection technique.

Additional requirements, if a set of "perfect" patterns is to be formed, are illustrated by the following:

d) Since the expected number of selections is 14.09, some of the patterns must have 15 selections and the sum of the probabilities of such patterns must be exactly .09.

ILLUSTRATION C
Worksheet for the formation of patterns for a controlled selection of hospitals

Pattern no.	1			2			...	n		
Pattern probability	.05			.08			...	.01		
Cumulative probability	.05			.13			...	1.00		
Geographic district	Type and size	Probability	Un-assigned prob.	Type and size	Probability	Un-assigned prob.	...	Type and size	Probability	Un-assigned prob.
1	2	3	4	2	3	4	...	2	3	4
I	M 4	.84	.79	M 5	.42	.34	...	M 3	.01	0
	M 6	.17	.12	M 4	.79	.71	...	M 5	.01	0
	—	—	—	—	—	—	...	O 4	.01	0
II	M 3	.50	.45	M 3	.45	.37	...	O 4	.01	0
	O 2	.50	.45	O 4	.45	.37	...	O 5	.01	0
	O 4	.50	.45	O 6	.08	.00	...			
III	M 3	.50	.45	M 4	.50	.42	...	M 3	.01	0
	M 5	.50	.45	M 6	.08	.00	...	M 4	.01	0
	O 4	.33	.28	—	—	—	...			
IV	M 2	.50	.45	M 2	.45	.37	...	M 2	.01	0
	M 4	.50	.45	O 4	.34	.26	...	M 5	.01	0
	O 5	.25	.20	M 5	.67	.59	...	O 6	.01	0
V	M 3	.75	.70	M 3	.70	.62	...	M 4	.01	0
	M 5	.50	.45	O 5	.08	.00	...	M 5	.01	0
VI	M 4	.66	.61	M 3	.50	.42	...	M 4	.01	0
	M 5	.50	.45	M 4	.61	.53	...	M 6	.01	0

Hospital size group and type*	Number of selections			
Size group				
2 (1.50)	2	1	...	1
3 (2.75)	3	3	...	2
4 (4.50)	5	5	...	5
5 (3.67)	4	3	...	4
6 (1.67)	1	2	...	2
Type				
Medical (10.51)	11	10	...	10
Osteo. (3.58)	4	4	...	4
Total (14.09)	15	14	...	14

* Numbers in parentheses are the expected numbers of selections (from Table 3).

Discussion of Illustration

The worksheet is used to record for each pattern the subclasses from which selections are to be made, the probabilities of selection for the patterns, and the cumulative probability over all patterns. It is convenient to record the pattern numbers on line 1 in the heading, the pattern probabilities on line 2, and the cumulative probability on line 3. The latter probability is derived by successive additions of the pattern probabilities. For example, both the first pattern probability and the first cumulative probability are .05; however, while the second pattern probability is .08, the cumulative probability is .05 + .08 = .13.

When ruling the midsection of the worksheet, allow as many lines for a district as the maximum number of selections to be made. This will help to keep the number of selections within the proper range. To illustrate, the expected number of noncertainty selections from district I is 2.72, from Table 3; hence, a pattern must include either two or three selections from the district, and a maximum of three lines is needed. In patterns 1 and 2, the dashes in the third line for district I denote that the omission of a third selection is intentional and not an oversight.

Cols. 2, 3 and 4 repeat for each pattern. Col. 2 identifies the selections by type and size group for each district. Col. 3 contains the available probabilities at any one stage of the selection

e) Continuing across the first line of Table 3, the probability of two selections from group 2 is .50; the probability of three from group 3 is .75; the probability of five (or of four) from group 4 is .50; the probability of four from 5 is .67 and the probability of two from 6 is .67.

Similar statements can be made for the state totals of medical and osteopathic hospitals, and then in turn for each district.

MAINTAINING OTHER CONTROL RECORDS

Not only must each pattern be recorded, but knowledge of the expected numbers remaining after the formation of each pattern is essential and available if a set of records is maintained for the total sample and for each district. This type of bookkeeping is illustrated and explained in Illustration D. After a pattern is formed, the appropriate probabilities are subtracted, cell by cell, throughout all record sheets. The sampler who devises a system of independent checks to detect clerical errors will be well repaid for his efforts. The selection procedure progresses smoothly if no errors are made, but it becomes tangled if they go unnoticed until final patterns are being formed. The last pattern should meet the same minimum requirements as the first. Although the formation of patterns which conform to the restrictions of the expected sample sizes is stressed, in some situations it may be more efficient to accept minor imperfections rather than revise substantial amounts of work.

CHOOSING ONE PATTERN FROM THE COMPLETED SET

Having completed a set of acceptable patterns, one is chosen at random. This the sampler accomplishes by resorting to a table of random numbers to obtain one within the range of 001 through 100 (assuming probabilities were computed to two decimals). Following along the cumulative probability line of Illustration C, he then locates the first cumulation equal to or greater than the random number; the pattern thus identified determines the number of selections from each of the noncertainty

---

procedure. In pattern 1 the col. 3 entries are taken from Table 3; beyond this point, the sampler is dependent upon his own record keeping. Col. 4 is obtained by subtracting the pattern probability from entries in col. 3. Thus, for pattern 1, col. 4 is col. 3 diminished by .05.

The pattern probability is arbitrarily chosen subject to the restraints of Table 3 and consistent with remaining expectations in Illustration D. The minimum value is .01; the maximum must not exceed the minimum value in col. 3. Pattern 1 probability may range from .01 through .17, and pattern 2 from .01 through .08. The decision to use the maximum possible probability per pattern or to choose a lesser value varies with technicians.

At the bottom of the worksheet a control is maintained on the total number of selections, by hospital size group and by type. Numbers in parentheses are the expectations, from Table 3. Having these figures for reference is an aid in maintaining an appropriate number of selections. For example, four selections from group 3 would be inconsistent with expectations, as would be only three selections from group 4. A pattern with nine medical and five osteopathic hospitals is unacceptable. (For further discussion see *Preparation of worksheet and formation of selection patterns* in the accompanying text.)

cells. These numbers of selections are combined with the certainty ones to give the total selections, cell by cell, for the sample. This is the source of the figures appearing as the actual sample in Table 2.

ILLUSTRATION D

Suggested control record for the total sample,* showing expected number of selections remaining after each pattern is subtracted

Pattern number		1	2	...	$n-1$	n
Pattern probability		.05	.08	...	x	.01
Cumulative probability		.05	.13	...	.99	1.00
Type and size group	Expected Number	Remaining Expectation	Remaining Expectation	...	Remaining Expectation	Remaining Expectation
M 2	1.00	.95	.87	...	.01	.00
M 3	2.50	2.35	2.11	...	.02	.00
M 4	3.00	2.85	2.61	...	.03	.00
M 5	2.67	2.52	2.36	...	.03	.00
M 6	1.34	1.29	1.21	...	.01	.00
O 2	.50	.45	.45	...	.00	.00
O 3	.25	.25	.25	...	.00	.00
O 4	1.50	1.40	1.24	...	.02	.00
O 5	1.00	.95	.87	...	.01	.00
O 6	.33	.33	.25	...	.01	.00
Total	14.09	13.34	12.22	...	.14	.00
Medical	10.51	9.96	9.16	...	.10	.00
Osteopathic	3.58	3.38	3.06	...	.04	.00
Number of Selections	*Probability*	*Unassigned Probability*	*Unassigned Probability*	...	*Unassigned Probability*	*Unassigned Probability*
Medical 10	.49	.49	.41	...	.01	.00
11	.51	.46	.46	...	.00	.00
Osteopathic 3	.42	.42	.42	...	.00	.00
4	.58	.53	.45	...	.01	.00
Total 14	.91	.91	.83	...	.01	.00
15	.09	.04	.04	...	.00	.00

* In addition, similar controls are recommended for *EACH* district.

Discussion of Illustration

In the first two columns are entered the possible combinations of type and size group with their respective expected number of selections, obtained from the totals in the second and third lines of Table 3. While the middle portion of the record keeps control of the expected number of selections, the lower portion checks on the probabilities of the specific numbers of selections. To illustrate, the expected number of medical hospitals is 10.51; therefore, the probability of having 11 selections is .51 and the probability of 10 selections is .49.

The entries for a pattern are made after an acceptable pattern has been developed. In fact, completing the control record may help to locate and prevent the use of unacceptable patterns. For example, there must be one M 2 selection in every pattern; there must be at least two M 3 selections in every pattern and 50 per cent of the time there must be three. The pattern entries are calculated by subtracting from the preceding column as many units of probability as have been used for the particular pattern, as illustrated:

For M 2: pattern 1 used 1 × 0.05. Therefore, the remainder is 1.00 − .05 = .95.
pattern 2 used 1 × 0.08. The remainder is 0.95 − .08 = .87.
For M 3: pattern 1 used 3 × 0.05. The remainder is 2.50 − .15 = 2.35.
Notice that after the $n-1$th pattern there remains an amount that will yield an acceptable pattern—no more and no less.

Selecting the Sample Hospitals Within Individual Cells

Now that the number of sample selections from each cell is known, how are these to be drawn? One answer is: at random from among the hospitals in the designated cells. On the other hand, the sampler may introduce further controls within the restrictions of specific substrata. This is the stage at which controls on ownership, accreditation, Blue Cross participation, and geographic location within districts were introduced (in addition to the controls on size, district, and hospital type). It is not necessary that the same controls or the same methods of control be used for every cell.

Since the hospitals with 250 to 499 beds are an important segment comprising nearly one-fourth of beds in the Michigan hospital universe, controls on ownership and geographic location across districts were given priority over control by district. However, controls on the selections of sample hospitals from the other size groups were maintained by district.

From Table 2 it can be seen that for the sample of hospitals in group 2, the following selections were to be made:

Type and District	No. in Univ.	No. in Sample
Medical		
I	3	1
II	8	4
Detroit city	4	2
Remainder of SMA	3	1
Remainder of district	1	1
III	4	2
IV	3	1
Osteopathic		
II	1	1
Total	19	9

Where one hospital is to be chosen from among three, selections can be made simultaneously with the drawing of one random number. The 2 in 4 selections may be obtained in a similar manner.

The patterns in Illustration E are three of several patterns acceptable with respect to size, ownership and geographic location. All medical hospitals in group 2 were accredited and all were Blue Cross-participating, obviating controls on these characteristics. A similar statement applies to Illustration F, with the qualification that there are two patterns instead of three.

With a larger investment in time, a controlled procedure could be developed for preferred combinations of the 1 in 3 (with probabilities of .33 each) and 1 in 2 (probabilities of .50 each) patterns.

With practice and experience the sampler acquires skill in developing control techniques and in judging which and how many controls are efficient. Where several selections are to be made from a cell and the

ILLUSTRATION E

Selecting a 1 in 3 sample of 250- to 499-bed hospitals in three districts, with controls by number of beds, ownership and city

District	PATTERNS								
	1			2			3		
	No. beds	Ownership	City	No. beds	Ownership	City	No. beds	Ownership	City
I	275	Church operated	a	305	Other nonprofit	b	294	Other nonprofit	a
II	366	City	c	348	City	d	278	Church operated	c
IV	291	Church operated	e	274	Other nonprofit	f	306	Church operated	f

ILLUSTRATION F

Selecting a 1 in 2 sample of 250- to 499-bed hospitals in two districts, with controls by number of beds, ownership, and city

DISTRICT	PATTERNS					
	1			2		
	No. beds	Ownership	City	No. beds	Ownership	City
II	401	Other nonprofit	g	396	Church operated	g
	270	Other nonprofit	g	305	Other nonprofit	g
III	341	Church operated	h	419	Other nonprofit	h
	253	Other nonprofit	i	320	Other nonprofit	h

sampling fraction does not combine easily with others, systematic selection with the appropriate sampling interval and a random start may be adequate after simple stratification by county and ownership, or perhaps by county, ownership and accreditation.

Illustration G demonstrates another procedure somewhat more complex, yet easily applied. Data on the number of district IV sample selections to be made and the number of hospitals in the universe, by size group and type, are from Table 2. Conveniently, eight is a common denominator for each of the sampling fractions. Thus within the probability requirements, the sampler may control the selection procedures with respect to the variables displayed in Illustration G, and make five selections with the choice of one random number. Capital and lower case letters designate hospitals and counties, respectively. When one hospital is to be selected from eight, each appears in one pattern, while if two selections are to be made, each hospital appears in two patterns. To satisfy the 1 in 2 selection, each hospital is assigned to four of the eight patterns. Although less apparent in the illustration, some gain in geographic spread among counties was achieved. Drawing at random within each cell could have resulted in five selections from only two counties (instead of four) and all of the same ownership (rather than three). Had not church-operated or church-related hospitals been assigned to different patterns, both hospitals of that ownership might have been selected, thus exaggerating that class of ownership in the sample.

COMPARISONS WITH THE UNIVERSE

The reader curious to know how closely the sample may be expected to reproduce the universe with respect to the control variables can form some general impressions from Table 4. To project the sample to the universe, a sample hospital's characteristics were weighted by the number of general beds in the hospital and then multiplied by the reciprocal of the hospital sampling fraction. The estimated number of beds formed the base of the sample proportions appearing in the table. Figures for the

ILLUSTRATION G
Controlled selection of hospitals in district IV, exclusive of size group 2

Size	Type	Number of sample selections from group	Hosp.	No. beds	Accredited	Ownership	Blue Cross	County
3	Medical	2 from 8	A	213	yes	Other nonprofit	yes	a
			B	207	"	" "	"	a
			C	192	"	" "	"	b
			✔D	177	"	" "	"	a
			E	175	"	" "	"	c
			F	160	"	" "	no	d
			✔G	121	"	" "	yes	e
			H	100	"	Church operated	"	b
4	Osteopathic	1 from 2	I	80	...	Other nonprofit	yes	f
			✔J	74	...	" "	"	a
5	Medical	1 from 8	K	48	no	" "	"	c
			L	44	"	" "	"	b
			M	43	yes	" "	"	g
			N	41	no	" "	"	e
			O	38	"	Church operated	"	h
			✔P	30	"	Proprietary	no	i
			Q	30	"	"	yes	j
			R	25	"	"	"	k
6	Medical	1 from 8	S	21	"	City	"	k
			✔T	20	no	"	"	b
			U	20	"	Proprietary	"	l
			V	20	"	"	"	l
			W	17	"	"	no	l
			X	16	"	"	"	m
			Y	14	"	"	yes	g
			Z	13	no	"	"	k

Pattern	group 3	group 4	group 5	group 6
1	B and C	I	K	X
2	G and D	J	L	S
3	E and F	J	M	Z
4	E and F	J	N	Y
5	B and C	I	O	W
✔6	G and D	J	P	T
7	A and H	I	Q	V
8	A and H	I	R	U

Checks (✔) identify the sample hospitals selected by randomly choosing pattern 6 from among the eight patterns.

universe are based on the complete count of general beds in hospitals with less than 500 beds.

The effective sample size for estimates in Table 4 is 39, the number of sample hospitals rather than the number of beds in sample hospitals. Furthermore, the sample is so constructed that sample hospitals represent roughly equal proportions of the universe. That is, each hospital represents about 1/39 of the universe. Therefore, in any classification, one sample hospital more or less can change the sample percentage from an overestimate to an underestimate of the comparable classification in the universe, and vice versa. For example, the sample estimates show 88 per cent of all beds are in medical hospitals and 12 per cent in osteopathic hospitals. If there had been one less osteopathic hospital in the sample and consequently one more medical hospital, the sample estimates might

TABLE 4—Per cent distribution of beds in hospitals with less than 500 beds, by selected characteristics of hospitals, for the universe and the sample; State of Michigan, 1958*

ITEM		Universe (per cent)	Sample (per cent)
Ownership or control		100	100
Government, nonfederal		16	15
Nonprofit		77	77
Church-operated or related	29		33
Other nonprofit	48		44
Proprietary		7	8
Blue Cross contracting		100	100
Participating		96	98
Nonparticipating		4	2
Type		100	100
Medical		90	88
Accredited	75		72
Nonaccredited	15		16
Osteopathic		10	12

* These universe figures were computed by first attributing the characteristics of a hospital to all general beds in the hospital, then computing the proportion of general beds associated with a specific characteristic. Symbolically, this is expressed as

$$P = \frac{\sum\limits_{g=2}^{6} \sum\limits_{h}^{M_g} \sum\limits_{i}^{B_{gh}} X_{ghi}}{\sum\limits_{g=2}^{6} \sum\limits_{h}^{M_g} B_{gh}}$$

Here P is a proportion.

X_{ghi} is to be associated with the ith bed in the hth hospital of the gth size group.

$X_{ghi} = 1$ if the ghth hospital belongs to classification X; if not, $X_{ghi} = 0$.

M_g is the number of hospitals in group g.

B_{gh} is the number of beds in the hth hospital of the gth group.

For all proportions the denominator is 21,290, the total number of general beds in all hospitals with less than 500 beds. (See Table 1, line 1.)

The estimates for the sample of 39 hospitals were made in a similar manner after weighting the number of general beds by the reciprocal of the sampling fraction for the sample hospitals. The expression for a sample estimate is

$$p = \frac{\sum\limits_{g=2}^{6} 1/f_g \sum\limits_{h}^{m_g} \sum\limits_{i}^{B_{gh}} X_{ghi}}{\sum\limits_{g=2}^{6} 1/f_g \sum\limits_{h}^{m_g} B_{gh}}$$

where m_g is the number of sample hospitals from the gth size group, f_g is the sampling fraction for the gth group, and other notations have the same interpretation as in the expression for P, the proportion in the universe. For all sample estimates the denominator is 21,046 which is an esimate of 21,290, the number of general beds in the universe of groups 2 through 6. The sample estimate differs from the universe value by about one per cent.

have been coincident with the figures of 90 per cent and 10 per cent shown for the universe. Part of the discrepancy arises from rounding error, for hospitals are regarded as units not to be divided for sampling purposes. If it were desirable to select 4.6 osteopathic hospitals rather than either 4 or 5, the sample figures in Table 4 might be in closer agreement with those for the universe.

Generally, all sample discharges from a hospital will not have identical values for important study variables, estimates will be less sensitive to a particular sample selection, and many sample estimates will approximate the universe figure more closely than do some in Table 4. However, it is possible that some estimates from the discharge study may deviate more widely from the population value. If the researcher desires a greater degree of reliability than might reasonably be expected from a sample of some specified size and on the basis of estimates similar to those in Table 4, he can increase the sample size, strengthen controls on the selection procedure, or alter the sample design.

Subsampling Hospitals

There were three research projects concerned with the study of institutions, as described in Chapter I:

1. Analysis of institutional accounting systems assessed in terms of agreement with accepted standards of good hospital and general accounting practices.
2. An inventory of institutional facilities and analysis of factors affecting their costs.
3. Study of external and internal controls affecting quantity, quality, and costs of health care administered in hospitals.

The basic sample of 47 hospitals used for the first study was supplemented (raising the total sample to 88 hospitals) for the second study and subsampled for the third. The purpose of this section is to illustrate a subsampling technique employed to reduce the core sample from 47 to 33 institutions.

The factors dictating the reduction in sample size for the "Control Study" centered around the objectives, nature of data collected, precision of estimates desired, expected variation in types of control in the various institutions, and limitations on time available for data collection. It was felt desirable to reduce the basic sample of 47 hospitals to around 30 by forming three size groups with approximately equal numbers of sample hospitals. One of the newly formed groups included hospitals with 100 through 499 beds.[4] In the original sample, nine institutions were selected at the rate of 1/2 from those with 250 to 499 beds, while 14 hospitals were selected from the 100- to 249-bed group which was sampled at the rate of 1/4. The samples from these two groups can be converted to a 1/6

---

[4] The other groups were: (1) hospitals with 500 or more beds; (2) hospitals with less than 100 beds. The eight large hospitals were included with certainty. A 1/12 sample of small hospitals was achieved by subsampling the 1/6 sample of hospitals with 50 to 99 beds, and supplementing the 1/24 sample of hospitals with less than 25 beds.

sample with controls by size, geographic location and ownership. Since each medical hospital was accredited and all were Blue Cross-participating, controls were unnecessary for these characteristics.

To change from a 1/2 to a 1/6 sample requires the elimination of two-thirds and the retention of one-third of the sample hospitals, while conversion from a 1/4 to a 1/6 sample is accomplished by eliminating one-third and retaining two-thirds of the original sample. The subsampling can be done simultaneously by forming preferred patterns such that, with respect to control variables, patterns I, II and III for the first group complement patterns I, II and III, respectively, of the second group. As shown in Illustration H, each hospital in the first group appears in only one pattern whereas each member of the second group appears in two patterns. The choice of one random number (1, 2 or 3) accomplished the subsampling at proper rates and satisfied the controls.

With this illustration, the description of hospital sampling is concluded. The next sampling problem confronting the investigator was that of sampling within hospitals.

ILLUSTRATION H
Controlled subselection of hospitals in two size groups of the Michigan sample

DISTRICT	HOSPITALS WITH 250–499 BEDS			HOSPITALS WITH 100–249 BEDS		
	Patterns			Patterns		
	I	II	III	I	II	III
	Hosp. and ownership codes[a]	Hosp. and ownership codes[a]	Hosp. and ownership codes[a]	Hosp. and ownership codes[a]	Hosp. and ownership codes[a]	Hosp. and ownership codes[a]
I	a 23			A 23 / B 13	A 23 / C 21	C 21 / B 13
II Detroit	b 23[b]	d 21	g 23	D 21 / E 23 / G 23 / H 21	E 23 / F 23 / G 23	D 21 / F 23 / H 21
Remainder of SMA		e 21			N 23[b]	N 23[b]
Remainder of district			h 21			
III		f 23	i 23	I 21	I 21	
IV	c 21			J 23	K 21	J 23 / K 21
V				L 21	L 21	
VI					M 13	M 13
Total number	3	3	3	9	10	9

[a] Lower case and capital letters identify hospitals in the two size groups, respectively; numbers to the right of letters are ownership codes:
   13 = county;   21 = church operated or church related;   23 = other nonprofit.
[b] Osteopathic hospitals; all others are medical.

THE SAMPLE OF DISCHARGES

Supplied with the patient sampling rates described earler in this chapter, one of two field teams visited each of the 47 hospitals and set about the task of obtaining the needed data for a sample of discharges from these hospitals during 1958. The over-all task was usually accomplished in six or seven stages:

1. determination of the type of record, or listing, to be used for sampling;
2. conversion of the listing to one of discharges from the hospital in 1958, if necessary;
3. application of the patient sampling rate to the listing and recording of basic identification information (name, medical record number, date of admission or discharge) for each selected hospital stay;
4. determination of the primary diagnosis for each selected patient stay;
5. subsampling those cases in the delivery and tonsils and adenoids categories, and cases in all categories other than the remaining sixteen chosen for intensive study;
6. augmentation of the samples from categories chosen for intensive study if deemed to be deficient (fewer than three cases);
7. transcription of the needed information (either basic demographic, diagnostic, and financial data or detailed clinical data, as set forth in Chapter I).

Several of these steps are described in detail.

Patient Lists Available for Sampling

The ease with which a list of discharges can be compiled depends upon the hospital system of record keeping. Many systems in current use proved to be "tailor-made" for sampling purposes, while others needed extensive conversion. What was sought in each hospital was a list of discharges (excluding newborn) in chronological order by date of discharge. Where this was present, and having determined that there was no evidence of cyclic effect, a random start was chosen (within the confines of the established interval) and the interval uniformly applied to all discharges during 1958. In those institutions where this type of record was not available, an attempt was made to emulate it. Other major sources for listings and the steps necessary for conversion follow.

The most common listing available was the admission ledger, or some variation on it. This record usually had all patients entered in chronological order by time of admission, along with name, age, sex, type of service (medical, surgical, obstetrical, pediatric, etc.), date of discharge, and name of admitting physician. This type of listing was converted to a listing of discharges by first omitting cases that were *not* discharged in 1958 (those cases discharged in 1959 or later) before applying the sampling interval. This resulted in a sample of those persons both admitted *and* discharged in 1958. This left the problem of identifying those patients who were admitted earlier than 1958 but discharged during the study period. A simple method of including these patients was to use the midnight census of December 31, 1957, employing the same interval as used for the 1958 admissions. However, the daily census was not available for all hospitals and an alternative method of sampling had to be found. A laborious, but satisfactory, procedure consisted of examining the ledger of earlier admissions and counting only those cases discharged in 1958. Fortunately, this latter procedure was necessary in only a few isolated instances.

In one hospital there was no master list of either admissions or discharges during the year. However, the medical records were filed by year. There it was necessary to assemble all records of all patients and order them chronologically by date of discharge before selecting the sample.

Some hospitals maintain a complete set of *daily* admission and discharge sheets instead of a single continuous listing of admissions or discharges in order by *time* of admission. Where patients are listed in order by time of admission or discharge *within* day of admission, the sampling procedure is straightforward. However, patients are sometimes ordered along some other factor (alphabetical order, type of service, name of physician, nursing unit, etc.) on these daily records. Here, in order to prevent any unknown bias, it was necessary to make a random selection within each interval. That is to say, patients were counted in the order listed on the sheets, the interval applied (say 8), a random number chosen (equal to or less than 8, but greater than zero), and the corresponding case selected.

Determination of Primary Diagnosis

Execution of one of the sampling procedures produced a list at the rate $1/n$ of discharges from a particular hospital during 1958. The next step was to determine the primary discharge diagnosis for each of these cases as a prelude to the patient subsampling procedures yet to be discussed.

In general, no single source outside of the medical record was found to give a consistently accurate account of the primary discharge diagnosis. In fact, the face sheet of the medical record itself, which usually contains a summary of the patient's disorders in order of importance, was found to be totally inadequate in a great number of cases. Most of the sample hospitals used a medical record face sheet which had separate sections for entering the admission diagnoses and discharge diagnoses. A frequent practice on the part of the attending physician was to write "same" in the discharge diagnosis section, apparently indicating that both the number and rank order of the diagnoses entered upon admission remained constant. However, it was discovered that in some cases although additional diagnoses were made or the rank order changed during the stay, the additions or changes were not entered on the face sheet. As a necessary precaution, therefore, the practice of scanning parts of the medical record (operation record, history, discharge notes, etc.) was instituted before categorizing the case according to diagnosis. It was the general impression of the field teams that this was a requisite to accurate categorization.

In a great many cases, primary diagnosis as a concept is simply ignored. In practice, diagnoses are listed in any order and some are included, others excluded on a hit-or-miss basis. In a majority of cases where only one diagnosis was listed (a common practice), that diagnosis was conceived of as primary in some sense.

Theoretically the concept of primary diagnosis is variously used and interpreted. In the first place, there is some feeling that this concept is clinically unsound and should not be used at all, the reason being that all diagnoses are important.

Where the concept is used, it may mean one of the following:

1. the diagnosis that is etiologically most basic;
2. the diagnosis that is most severe in implications for the patient (most disabling, most dangerous, poorest prognosis);
3. the diagnosis which occasions most of the treatment during the hospital stay;
4. the diagnosis which precipitates the particular hospital admission selected in the sample.

The last of these four meanings was chosen as the easiest to determine and the best suited for a study of hospital use. In actual fact, without regard to theory, by instinct, default, or for whatever reason, this is also the definition implied in the selection of a primary or a single diagnosis for listing by most of the physicians in the records studied. It should be apparent that the discharge diagnosis is less tentative and more definitive than the admitting diagnosis. The latter is often necessarily little more than an educated guess.

Subsampling Diagnostic Categories

In choosing the over-all patient sampling rate of 1/48, it was expected that there would be a surfeit of cases in the most frequently appearing diagnostic categories. An early decision was made to subsample those particular categories in order to reduce the costs of field work and data processing.

In each hospital a double sampling device was used. First, the originally selected cases were listed by diagnosis in chronological order; then cases not included in the 18 categories chosen for intensive analysis were subsampled at the rate of 1/3. Within the 18 categories, deliveries were subsampled at the rate of 1/10 and cases in the tonsils and adenoids category at 1/3, choosing appropriate random starts and applying the respective intervals. The savings in costs of field work produced by employing this subsampling routine outweighed the savings in analysis inherent in a self-weighting sample as originally considered.

Augmentation

With the listing, determination of primary diagnoses and subsampling complete, the teams counted the cases in each of the 18 diagnostic categories chosen for intensive study. If there were fewer than three cases in any one category, this number was augmented to three. Since it was not anticipated that any category would require augmentation in every hospital, it was thought that a minimum of three in a deficient category would yield about 200 cases in all for each low-frequency diagnosis.

To supplement the number of cases selected in a sample hospital, the 1958 universe of cases in the particular diagnostic category was first determined; then cases already selected were excluded. Based on the number of cases needed, a proper sampling interval was calculated, the additional cases selected, and their medical records abstracted. The determination of the universe was the difficult part of this process.[5] The most useful single source for counting the universe of cases was the hospital's diagnostic index.

Many hospitals maintain card files or ledgers, or lists recording case number, dates of admission and discharge and the diagnosis or diagnoses, either by name or by code number. Two systems of coding are in general use—the Standard Nomenclature of Diseases and Operations, and the International Statistical Classification of Diseases, Injuries and Causes of Death. Many hospitals, particularly smaller ones, use simplified or modified versions of these systems.

The categories of the Standard Nomenclature are minutely detailed, being coded first according to the site of the disease and then by its etiology. It was necessary to add together many of these classifications to constitute one of the study's diagnostic categories, such as appendicitis, and especially such broader categories as urinary tract infection or conditions of pregnancy.

The International Classification, with its more inclusive codes, designed particularly for research purposes, was easier to use. Some hospitals used modifications of older systems, or used their own unique systems.

Regardless of the nomenclature or coding, diagnostic indexes were of

---

[5] That is, not only the size of the universe but also the identity, by case number, of its constituent members.

three types—simple, multiple, and cross-indexed. The simple indexing listed the case under the primary diagnosis only; the multiple listed the case under *each* recorded diagnosis (i.e., the case number and hospitalization dates appeared on two to eight or more different file cards in different locations); the cross-index gave the code number of all other diagnoses with the case number on each diagnostic card where the case was listed.

In the latter two systems, it was generally impossible to determine which diagnosis was primary. Therefore, a slightly higher number of cases was sought, and the cases in which the given diagnosis was not primary were dropped after examination of the medical records, and no replacement was made.[6]

Two hospitals had diagnostic indexes coded and punched on IBM cards. Each coded the primary diagnosis as such, and according to the definition of primary diagnosis used in this study. Needless to say, this simplified the task considerably.

A number of hospitals were PAS members and had six-month summaries of all discharges, segregated by primary diagnosis, with other diagnoses and operations coded as cross-references. These lists, compiled for each member hospital in PAS, were ideally suited to the purposes of this study. In addition to card files, IBM cards and PAS data summaries, diagnostic indexes were kept in one other form—a book or ledger with pages or sections allotted to each diagnostic heading, listing case numbers and hospitalization dates.

In some hospitals no diagnostic indexes were kept. In others the indexes were so far out of date, incomplete, inaccurate, or otherwise inadequate that they could not be used. In these hospitals, admission or discharge ledgers were used, provided that they listed the final (as opposed to admitting) and primary diagnoses. In one hospital, all of the medical records for the year were used for both the original sampling and the augmentation in the absence of any adequate central access system.

To select cases for augmentation, the sampling interval was calculated from the total number in the universe and the number of additional cases needed, and an appropriate random number was selected. The sampling followed methods similar to those employed to select the initial patient sample. If the cases were not already in chronological order by date of discharge, as they were most of the time, they were so ordered before sampling.

SUMMARY

In this chapter, a probability design for a sample of general hospitals and patients was presented and illustrated with a description of a sample

---

[6] Cases selected in the original sample   0   1   2   3
Additional cases needed   3   2   1   0
Cases selected to allow for nonprimary diagnosis   4   3   2   0
In most cases these numbers sufficed, but in no case was the augmentation process repeated.

of 47 hospitals selected for the Michigan *Study of Hospital and Medical Economics*.

Using the technique of controlled selection, hospitals were selected while controlling on size, type, geographic area, and, with less stringency, ownership, Blue Cross participation, and accreditation; this technique permitted the selection of a relatively small number of hospitals which reproduced the universe well.

Discharges from general hospitals were sampled in such a manner that the product of the two sampling fractions, first for hospitals and second for discharges, was a basic 1 in 48 sample of all discharges from Michigan general hospitals during 1958. Infrequently appearing diagnostic categories were augmented and large, frequently appearing categories were subsampled. Consequently, the sample was no longer self-weighting, and each sample case was assigned a specific weight reflecting its probability of selection.

Chapter IV

Estimation Procedures

The decision to use a probability sample for the Michigan study of discharges developed from the need and desire to produce, from sample data, figures that would be characteristic not of discharges from some 40 or 50 hospitals but of discharges from all general hospitals in the state. To be valid, estimates must be calculated according to mathematical formulas which take into consideration the selection procedures and probabilities. Appropriately, estimation formulas are part of the sample design. Since this statement applies to estimates derived from samples of institutions as well as to samples of patients, some estimation techniques for each sample will be described.

For the Sample of Patients

The sample of patients was designed to estimate ratios (means or proportions) and comparisons or differences between ratios [21]. Although the sample was not expected to yield precise estimates of aggregates, in the analysis it was desirable to make limited use of this type of estimate also. Each of the three kinds of estimates is illustrated in Chapter V. The percentages in Tables 5, 7 and 11, and the averages in Tables 6, 8, 9, 10, and 12 are forms of ratio estimates. Tables 8, 9 and 10 also show comparisons between ratios while estimates of the number of discharges by hospital size group appear in Table 12. The estimation formulas which follow are generalizations of those used to prepare Tables 5 through 12.

The ratio estimator is of the form

$$r = y/x = \sum_{g}^{L} \sum_{h}^{m_g} y_{gh} \Big/ \sum_{g}^{L} \sum_{h}^{m_g} x_{gh} , \qquad (1)$$

where

$$y_{gh} = \sum_{i}^{n_{gh}} w_{ghi}\, y_{ghi} .$$

That is, y_{ghi} is one of the n_{gh} individual observations in the ghth hospital, and the observation is weighted by w_{ghi}. Similarly,

$$x_{gh} = \sum_{i}^{n_{gh}} w_{ghi}\, x_{ghi} .$$

m_g is the number of sample hospitals selected from the gth size group.[1]
L is the number of size groups.[1]

---

[1] When research is conducted in only one hospital, both m_g and L have values of 1.

If a constant over-all sampling fraction is used, $w_{ghi} = 1$. However, if disproportionate sampling is employed, appropriate weights inversely proportional to the probability of selection are required to avoid bias.[2]

The variate x is commonly the unit of analysis or element (for example, discharges) in the survey design; in this case r is the mean of the variate y per x element. This type of estimate is illustrated by the average length of stay of 7.4 days (Table 6) for all discharges. Very often y is a binomial variate such that y denotes the subclass of x with a specific characteristic, and r denotes the proportion of x possessing the characteristic (Table 7).

Two ratios, r_1 and r_2 may be compared by observing their difference, $r_1 - r_2$ (Table 8); or there may be interest in the difference between two aggregates, $Y_1' - Y_2'$. Such comparisons are common between two subgroups of the population.

The size groups and the geographic districts are special classes of subgroups for which the preceding estimates may be desirable and meaningful, providing the number of primary selections is sufficiently large, perhaps six or more. To illustrate, in Table 5 separate estimates for the first four size groups are derived from samples of eight or more hospitals yielding samples of discharges large enough for separate estimates of a number of characteristics, most appropriately in the form of proportions. In contrast, groups 5 and 6 were combined since neither of these groups had samples adequate for separate estimates.

In the expression $r = y/x$, y and x are the sample totals or convenient multiples of the sample totals (see footnote 2). To estimate, by expansion of the sample, the population aggregates Y and X, it is necessary to multiply the sample totals by the reciprocal of the over-all sampling fraction, f. Thus, $Y' = y/f$ and $X' = x/f$.

---

[2] To satisfy multiple objectives, the Michigan sample of discharges deviated from a self-weighting sample in several respects. The weighting scheme described below is a simplified version of the one actually used.

1. Delivery cases from the 1 in 48 sample were subsampled at the rate of 1 in 10. For this group the weight was 480.

2. Diagnostic categories exclusive of those discussed in 3, below, were a 1 in 3 subsample of the 1 in 48 selections. Here the weight was 144.

3. Categories selected for intensive study were supplemented at varying rates to yield sufficient sample sizes. The formulation of the weighting scheme to utilize all information was

$$\text{weight} = \frac{1}{f_g}\left(\frac{1}{f_{gh}}\right), \text{ where } f_{gh} = \frac{n_{ghd}}{N_{ghd}},$$

and

f_g is the sampling fraction for hospitals in the gth size group.
f_{gh} is the sampling fraction of discharges within hospitals in the gth size group.
N_{ghd} is the total number of cases in universe of the dth diagnostic category in the ghth hospital.
n_{ghd} is the total number of sample cases selected from the dth diagnostic category in the ghth hospital.

To simplify the processing of data, an adjusted constant sampling fraction, f, was determined in such a manner that $w_{ghi} = 1$ for *all* sample cases (whether class 1, 2 or 3 above or the 1/48 selections) and $f = 1/4.848$. In the tabulations, then, the data were self-weighting.

FOR A SAMPLE OF INSTITUTIONS

When the unit of analysis is the institution and the number of sample hospitals from a group is large enough for reliable estimates, a useful estimate is the mean per hospital,

$$\bar{y}_g = \frac{y_g}{m_g}. \tag{3}$$

Here $y_g = \overset{m_g}{\underset{h}{\Sigma}} y_{gh}$, where y_{gh} is the observed value of characteristic y for

the hth hospital in group g; m_g is the number of sample hospitals. No weighting is necessary because each hospital has equal weight within the size group. However, to estimate the aggregate Y_g' for the hospitals of group g, the appropriate weight is $1/f_g$, where f_g is the sampling fraction for hospitals in the gth group. That is,

$$Y_g' = \frac{y_g}{f_g}. \tag{4}$$

Whenever an average over size groups is desired, the $\bar{y}_g$ should be weighted in proportion to their contribution to or effect on the state total. Number of beds is suggested as a measure of this effect since a hospital with 700 beds, for example, has the capacity or opportunity to serve roughly seven times as many patients as a hospital with 100 beds. A weighted average or mean is then

$$\bar{y} = \overset{L}{\underset{g}{\Sigma}} B_g \, \bar{y}_g \bigg/ \overset{L}{\underset{g}{\Sigma}} B_g = \frac{1}{B} \overset{L}{\underset{g}{\Sigma}} B_g \, \bar{y}_g \,, \tag{5}$$

where B_g is the total number of beds for all hospitals in group g, B is $\overset{L}{\underset{g}{\Sigma}} B_g$, and L is the number of size groups.

The estimates described here are by no means exhaustive. The researcher may have interest in and need for other estimation techniques [2, 18], or he may seek counsel from a specialist to solve particular problems of estimation.

Chapter V
Sampling Variability

Estimates of the characteristics of hospitals and of patients are subject to error because only some of the hospitals and some of the records are included in a study. Although sampling is not the only source of error, it is the only type of error readily estimated from the sample.[1]

Procedures for estimating the sampling variability of cluster samples (generally, the patients of a hospital comprise a cluster) can be found in the literature [2, 18, 21]. However, estimation techniques adjusted to the sample design and to the specific estimates of the preceding section may be easier for the nontechnician to follow. As a matter of convenience the formulas for approximating the sampling error are in terms of the variance, the square of the standard error.

In order that the estimates of sampling variability may be calculated, it is necessary in the data collection stage that each hospital have a unique code and that each observation be coded with respect to the hospital of origin. Later, additional codes may be assigned to the hospitals selected with certainty and codes reassigned in a meaningful order to the hospitals in the other groups.

For the Sample of Patients

An approximation to the variance of the ratio estimator $r = y/x$ from equation (1), is

$$\text{var}(r) \doteq \frac{1}{x^2} \left[\text{var}(y) + r^2 \, \text{var}(x) - 2r \, \text{cov}(y, x) \right] ,$$

where "var" is to be read as "variance of" and "cov" read as "covariance of."

Two separate techniques are suggested: one for the hospitals selected with certainty and the other for hospitals selected with probability less than 1. The formulations are illustrated in terms of the Michigan sample. The expression for the sampling variability of r can be simplified by rewriting equation (1) as

$$r = y/x = \left(\sum_{h}^{8} y_h + \sum_{h'}^{39} y_{h'} \right) \bigg/ \left(\sum_{h}^{8} x_h + \sum_{h'}^{39} x_{h'} \right). \tag{1'}$$

This formula expresses the sample total y as the sum of the observations

---

[1] There may be errors in transcription, coding, processing, or tabulating. Lack of uniformity in designation of primary diagnosis is one source of nonsampling error. See Chapter III for a discussion of the concept of primary diagnosis and difficulties encountered in determining this from hospital medical records.

from two stratum groups: the eight Michigan hospitals selected with certainty, plus the sum of the observations from the 39 noncertainty hospitals. A similar statement applies to the total for x. The subscripts h and h' identify the two stratum groups.

Hospitals Selected with Certainty

Sampling variability arises among this group because of the sampling of patients within each hospital. The total variation within a hospital may be estimated by contrasting a proper one-half selection of the sample elements with the other one-half.[2] By creating two half-samples within each of the eight Michigan hospitals, 16 groups were formed and numbered so that numbers 1 and 2 were assigned to one hospital, 3 and 4 to another, and so on. The square of the difference between sample totals for members of a pair is the contribution from that hospital to the total variance of a characteristic y. The expressions for the variance of y, the variance of x and the covariance of y and x are respectively,

$$\sum_{h}^{8} (y_{h_1} - y_{h_2})^2 , \sum_{h}^{8} (x_{h_1} - x_{h_2})^2 , \sum_{h}^{8} (y_{h_1} - y_{h_2}) (x_{h_1} - x_{h_2}) ,$$

where y_{h_1}, y_{h_2}, x_{h_1}, and x_{h_2} are the half-sample totals for the hth hospital, and the summations are over the eight hospitals.

Hospitals Selected with Probability Less Than 1

Several estimation techniques are available [21], but only one will be discussed briefly. The particular method is that of successive differences from a systematic ordering of hospitals by size group and geographic location, and type within groups. For the Michigan sample each of the 39 hospitals was assigned a number in sequence once the ordering had been determined.[3] The approximations for the variances of y and x, and for the covariance of y and x are

$$\frac{39}{76} \sum_{h'}^{38} (y_{h'} - y_{h'+1})^2 , \quad \frac{39}{76} \sum_{h'}^{38} (x_{h'} - x_{h'+1})^2 ,$$

and

$$\frac{39}{76} \sum_{h'}^{38} (y_{h'} - y_{h'+1}) (x_{h'} - x_{h'+1}) .$$

---

[2] This was done by assigning the first, third, etc., selections of patients to one half-sample and sample patients two, four, etc., to the other half-sample.

[3] Beginning with size group 2, the medical hospitals were ordered by geographic district (I through IV since there were no hospitals of this size in V or VI) and then followed with the osteopathic hospital. Continuing into group 3, and starting with the osteopathic hospital, the ordering then proceeded with medical hospitals from districts I through VI, then was reversed with group 4, going from medical hospitals in group VI to group I. The process was continued till each of the 39 hospitals had been ordered.

The Total Sample

Combining the estimates for the two stratum groups (the certainty and the noncertainty hospitals) the variance estimate for the total sample is

$$
\text{var}(r) \doteq \frac{1}{x^2} \left\{ \sum_{h}^{8} (y_{h_1} - y_{h_2})^2 + \frac{39}{76} \sum_{h'}^{38} (y_{h'} - y_{h'+1})^2 \right.
$$

$$
+ r^2 \left[\sum_{h}^{8} (x_{h_1} - x_{h_2}) + \frac{39}{76} \sum_{h'}^{38} (x_{h'} - x_{h'+1})^2 \right]
$$

$$
\left. - 2r \left[\sum_{h}^{8} (y_{h_1} - y_{h_2})(x_{h_1} - x_{h_2}) + \frac{39}{76} \sum_{h'}^{38} (y_{h_1'} - y_{h_2'})(x_{h_1'} - x_{h_2'}) \right] \right\}. \quad (6)
$$

This computation is valid for any mean or proportion.

The multiplier $(1-f)$, sometimes referred to as the finite population correction [2, p. 17], has been omitted because its value is generally close to 1 for samples of patients and consequently has little effect on the final result; if the effect of the multiplier is significant, it should be included.

The variance of an aggregate $Y' = y/f$ may be derived from the expression for the variance of y given in equation (6). Thus,

$$
\text{var}(Y') = \frac{1}{f^2} [\text{var}(y)] = \frac{1}{f^2} \left[\sum_{h}^{8} (y_{h_1} - y_{h_2})^2 + \frac{39}{76} \sum_{h'}^{38} (y_{h'} - y_{h'+1})^2 \right]. \quad (7)
$$

To estimate the variance of the difference between two ratios r_1 and r_2, one needs to know the variance of each and in addition their covariance. The general form of the estimate is

$$
\text{var}(r_1 - r_2) = \text{var}(r_1) + \text{var}(r_2) - 2\text{cov}(r_1, r_2). \quad (8)
$$

The variance of each ratio can be estimated from equation (6). An estimate of the covariance is

$$
\text{cov}(r_1, r_2) \doteq \frac{1}{x_1 x_2} [\text{cov}(y_1, y_2) + r_1 r_2 \text{cov}(x_1, x_2) - r_2 \text{cov}(y_1, x_2) - r_1 \text{cov}(y_2, x_1)]. \quad (9)
$$

In the notation of equation (6), the covariance of y_1 and y_2 for the Michigan sample becomes

$$
\text{cov}(y_1, y_2) \doteq \sum_{h}^{8} (y_{1h_1} - y_{1h_2})(y_{2h_1} - y_{2h_2}) + \frac{39}{76} \sum_{h'}^{38} (y_{1h'} - y_{1h'+1})(y_{2h'} - y_{2h'+1}). \quad (10)
$$

Similar expansions may be made for the other three covariance terms of equation (9).

The variance of the difference between aggregates is similar in form to equation (8); that is,

$$
\text{var}(Y_1' - Y_2') = \text{var}(Y_1') + \text{var}(Y_2') - 2 \text{cov}(Y_1', Y_2'). \quad (11)
$$

When Y_1' and Y_2' are estimated from the same sample,

$$
\text{var}(Y_1' - Y_2') = \frac{1}{f^2} [\text{var}(y_1) + \text{var}(y_2) - 2 \text{cov}(y_1, y_2)]. \quad (12)
$$

For a Sample of Institutions

The variance of the estimate

$$\bar{y}_g = \frac{y_g}{m_g} \tag{3}$$

may be approximated by

$$\text{var}(\bar{y}_g) \doteq \frac{(1 - f_g)}{2m_g (m_g - 1)} \sum_{h}^{m_g - 1} (y_{gh} - y_{gh+1})^2 , \tag{13}$$

where y_{gh} is the observed value for the hth hospital and m_g the number of sample hospitals in the gth group. Notice that the variance estimate appropriately becomes zero for a group with $f_g = 1$; that is, when all hospitals in the group have been included with certainty, there is no sampling variability.

The aggregate $Y_g' = y_g/f_g$ (4)

can also be expressed as $\dfrac{m_g}{f_g} \bar{y}_g$, where m_g/f_g is a constant. Then the variance of Y_g' can be estimated as

$$\text{var}(Y_g') = [m_g^2 / f_g^2] \text{ var}(\bar{y}_g) . \tag{14}$$

Now, regarding the samples among size groups as independent, the variance of

$$\bar{y} = \frac{1}{B} \sum_{g}^{L} B_g \bar{y}_g \tag{5}$$

can be estimated from

$$\text{var}(\bar{y}) = \frac{1}{B^2} \sum_{g}^{L} B_g^2 [\text{var}(\bar{y}_g)] . \tag{15}$$

As in Chapter IV, B_g is the number of beds in all hospitals of size group g, and B is the sum of beds in the universe of hospitals.

Some Empirical Results

The efficacy of the Michigan sample may be appraised by calculating and examining estimates of sampling variability, or by comparing sample estimates with comparable independent estimates or with known values for the universe. It is appropriate to inquire: Does the sample provide acceptable estimates for the universe of hospital discharges? How well does it reflect the range of diagnostic categories for all hospitals and for the several size groups? What recommendations can be made for future samples of hospitals and patients? Response to these and similar questions can be made in reference to the sample of discharges selected for the study of the "Character and Effectiveness of Hospital Use," this being the only study for which calculations of sampling variability have been completed. The presentation of these data serves a dual purpose: to provide bases for evaluating the quality of the sample; and to make available for use in the planning of future studies this sampling experience within a new subject area.

Comments are restricted to sampling error or variability, with only brief remarks on nonsampling errors and biases which may be important also. These include, for example, nonresponse, transcription and processing errors, incomplete and inadequate records, error or bias in abstraction of records. Nonresponse is interpreted as failure to gain cooperation, and hence access to records, from a sample hospital. Of 47 hospitals selected for the Michigan study, one was unable to cooperate because of extensive remodeling at the time of investigation, and a substitution was made from the same cell (size, geographic area, hospital type) of the universe. This departure from probability sampling introduces an unknown bias which in some degree affects each sample estimate, including those of sampling variability. In considering alternatives, substitution was preferred to the weighting of responses to compensate for nonresponse. Investigation into the effects of nonresponse has not been undertaken nor is measurement of other nonsampling errors or biases under study at present.

Sampling Variability of Estimates

The quality of sample estimates is to be evaluated relative to intended use. Estimates adequate for some purposes are inadequate for others. The measures of sampling variability presented in Tables 5 through 11 enable the reader to judge if this sample meets his standards or in what ways it fails, thus indicating opportunities for improvements in design. The detail of Table 5 permits comparisons among hospital size groups with respect to diagnostic categories, while Tables 6 through 11 display data relating to lengths of stay, sources of payment, and utilization of laboratory procedures. (Data in Tables 6 through 11 appear also in the study report.)

The percentages and means were calculated from equation (1)[4]. Estimates of sampling variability were computed from equation (6) for

---

[4] The percentages by size group in Table 5 were computed from

$$r_g = y_g / x_g = \sum_h^{m_g} \sum_i^{n_{gh}} w_{ghi} \, y_{ghi} \bigg/ \sum_h^{m_g} \sum_i^{n_{gh}} w_{ghi} \, x_{ghi} \,,$$

where m_g, the number of sample hospitals, has the values of 8, 9, 14, 10, and 6, respectively. This expression differs from equation (1) only in that the summation over the five size groups is omitted because each is considered individually.

means and percentages,[5] and from appropriate adaptations of equations (8) and (10) for the estimated differences in Tables 8, 9 and 10.

In each table approximate standard errors of estimates are displayed.[6] If the sampling process were repeated many times under the same conditions, some of the samples would yield estimates larger than the population value and some estimates would be smaller. The standard error is a measure of this chance fluctuation due to sampling. It does not measure the actual error of a particular sample estimate; it leads to statements in the form of confidence intervals that are correct in a specified proportion of cases in the long run. In about 68 cases out of 100, a range of one standard error on either side of a sample estimate can be expected to include the population value. In about 95 cases out of 100 the population value will be included within a range defined by two standard errors on either side of a sample estimate.

Consider the estimated average length of hospital stay for all diagnoses; in Table 6 the estimate is shown to be 7.4 days, with an approximate standard error of .2 days. It is not known if the estimate is larger or smaller than the value that would have been obtained if *all* rather than a sample of discharges had been included in the study. It is likely that the range 7.2 to 7.6 days (i.e., 7.4 ± .2) includes the population value, and it is even more probable that the true value lies within the range 7.0 to 7.8 days. If one requires a greater degree of confidence the range may be widened.[7]

Generally, the precision of sample estimates can be raised by increasing the sample size either of hospitals or patients, or by some combination of these. Conversely, if less precision is acceptable, some savings may be effected by reducing the sample size or changing the design.

---

[5] Estimates of sampling variability by size group in Table 5 were derived from equation (6) and adapted to each size group separately. For the eight hospitals of group 1,

$$r = \sum_h^8 \sum_i^{n_h} w_{hi} y_{hi} \bigg/ \sum_h^8 \sum_i^{n_h} w_{hi} x_{hi},$$

and

$$\text{var}(r) \doteq \frac{1}{\left(\sum_h^8 \sum_i^{n_h} w_{hi} x_{hi}\right)^2} \sum_h^8 \left[(y_{h_1} - y_{h_2}) - r(x_{h_1} - x_{h_2})\right]^2 .$$

Here g is omitted from the notation, since it has the value of 1. For the remaining groups

$$\text{var}(r_g) \doteq \frac{1}{\left(\sum_h \sum_i w_{ghi} x_{ghi}\right)^2} \cdot \frac{m_g}{2(m_g - 1)} \sum_{h'}^{m_g - 1} \left[(y_{gh'} - y_{gh'+1}) - r_g(x_{gh'} - x_{gh'+1})\right]^2 ,$$

where m_g has the values 9, 14, 10 and 6, respectively, for groups 2, 3, 4, and 5 and 6 combined.

[6] The IBM 704 program used in the calculations of sampling variability was developed by the Survey Research Center's Sampling Section and the Statistical Analysis Section of the Institute for Social Research.

[7] The reader is referred to the literature for more extended discussions of the interpretation of the standard error [7, pp. 449–54; 18, pp. 20–34; 32, pp. 190–6; 27].

Estimates of sampling variability are themselves affected by chance fluctuations which may be substantial particularly for estimates derived from small numbers of hospitals or patients, or both. Therefore, sampling errors presented in the tables are to be regarded as approximate rather than exact values.

INTERPRETING TABLE 5

Only cursory treatment of this table is possible here, since complete comprehension of the data requires more extensive analyses than have been accomplished. For the state as well as for five hospital size groups, Table 5 presents four values for each of 35 diagnostic categories: (1) the estimated per cent of hospitalizations attributed to a particular diagnostic category; (2) the standard error of the estimated per cent; (3) the ratio of the sample variance (square of the standard error) to the variance that would be experienced under assumptions of simple random sampling; (4) the actual number of sample cases from which estimates were derived. Earlier discussions of techniques used to estimate the per cents and their standard errors are not repeated here. Generally, these two measures will satisfy the purposes of readers less technically oriented, while those concerned with sample design and sampling variability among hospital size groups may be interested in the comparisons of variances and in numbers of sample cases by diagnostic category.

The variance of simple random sampling serves as a standard with which comparisons can be made to evaluate the precision of alternate designs [18, pp. 259, 401] or to contrast sampling variability among hospital size groups. The ratio of the sample variance to that of simple random sampling was obtained for each estimated per cent by first computing the sample variance according to formulas presented earlier (equations (6), (8), (10) and footnote 5), then dividing the sample variance by the variance associated with a per cent (p) obtained from a simple random sample of the same size (n) as the Michigan sample. An illustration will clarify this explanation.

In the hospitals with 500 or more beds, approximately 4.5 per cent of all discharges had primary diagnoses in the malignant neoplasm category (Table 5, column 6). The variance of this estimate is .25, obtained by squaring the standard error of .5 per cent (from column 7). Now, the total number, n, of sample cases in the large hospitals was 1,585. Assuming the estimated per cent, $p = 4.5$, resulted from a simple random sample of 1,585 cases, the simple random variance (srv) would be

$$\text{srv} = p(1-p)/n = 4.5(95.5)/1{,}585 = .27$$

and $\qquad$ sample variance/srv $= .25/.27 = 0.9,$

which appears in column 8 as the ratio of variances.

Ratios less than one indicate the sample design produced more precise estimates than would have been obtained from a simple random sample of the same size, while ratios greater than one denote more sampling variability than with simple random sampling. As is the situation with other sample estimates, these ratios of variances are also subject to sampling variability. Stratification and controlled selection probably account for much of the reduction in sampling variability in the Michigan design, whereas clustering by hospital and some departures from a self-weighting sample would tend to increase sampling variation.

Sampling variability, expressed by the ratio of the sample variance to simple random variance, shows inverse relationship with size of hospital. Inasmuch as all of the large hospitals (500 or more beds) were included in the sample, sampling variability arises in this group because of the sampling within hospitals; therefore, estimates of proportions of discharges by diagnosis entail only small variations, although for other characteristics sampling error may increase. In the hospitals under 500 beds, sampling variability comes from two major sources: variation among hospitals and variation among patients within hospitals. Comparisons with simple random variances (columns 12, 16 and 20) indicate that, in general, the ranges of the ratios in size groups 2, 3, and 4 are not strikingly different. Looking next at the group of small hospitals, the comparisons of the sample variances with those of simple random sampling (column 24) show somewhat higher ratios than had been anticipated. From limited investigation it appears that the character of small hospitals is affected by geographic location. A small hospital in a large city may perform services quite different from those provided by a small community hospital. If true, this speaks well for control on both geographic area and hospital size.

Examination of the distributions of diagnoses by hospital size group suggests some clues to sources of variability affecting state estimates as well as those for individual groups. The data support what might have been anticipated. Diagnoses resulting in patient utilization of specialized treatments and medical skills, as in the case of malignant neoplasms, are more prevalent in large hospitals and decline in frequency with hospital size. Deliveries, tonsils and adenoids, and appendicitis, for examples, occur with greater relative frequency as hospital size decreases. Bronchopneumonia and other diseases of the respiratory system show some concentrations among smaller hospitals. However, this may be a geographic phenomenon occurring in areas serviced by smaller hospitals rather than being characteristic of small hospitals in general.

TABLES 6 THROUGH 11

Data in these tables relate to discharges from all general hospitals. The preceding discussions of sampling errors together with the illustrations which follow provide explanations adequate for general review and statistical interpretation of the data. For social and economic implications the reader is referred to the study report [11].

Table 6 presents the average (mean) length of stay for each of 35 diagnostic categories, the standard errors of the means, the coefficients of variation, and the number of sample cases on which each mean is based. The estimated means and their standard errors were calculated from equations (1) and (6) respectively. The coefficient of variation, which is the ratio of the standard error to the mean, is a measure of variability permitting comparisons among the 35 diagnostic categories. Most of the coefficients are within the range .03 to .1. As might be anticipated, their magnitudes show an inverse relationship to sample size, the highest coefficients occurring when the mean is based on fewer than 50 sample cases.

Table 7, which relates to primary source of payment, includes the four types of data encountered in Table 5—estimated per cents, standard errors of per cents, comparisons of sample variances with those of simple random sampling, and number of sample cases. The large ratios to simple random sampling (column 4) reflect the high degree of clustering by source of payment and demonstrate the inefficiency of the design if estimates of this characteristic were the primary consideration. If source of payment were the only interest, the information could be obtained with the same precision from a simple random sample of about 650 discharges. However, a sample of 650 would not yield sufficient numbers of discharges in many of the diagnostic categories; moreover, simple random samples are often impractical because a complete listing of the universe is unavailable for sampling.

Data in Tables 8 and 9 relate to hospital charges and average lengths of stay, respectively, by primary source of payment. The construction of the tables is similar to that of Table 6. However, in addition to means and their sampling variability, Tables 8 and 9 display differences between pairs of means and the sampling errors of comparisons. Consider, in Table 8, the comparison of average total hospital charges when Blue Cross-Blue Shield and commercial insurance are primary sources of payment. The difference in charges is estimated to be $42, and the approximate standard error is $10. The chances are about 95 in 100 that the "true" difference is between $22 and $62—that is, a range of $20 on either side of the estimated difference. The probability that the "true" difference could be zero (that is, more than four standard errors below the estimate of $42) is too small for practical consideration. On the other hand, when commercial insurance and the patient are compared as primary sources of payment, total hospital charges differ by about $19 and the standard error is nearly $10. While the odds are against a "true" difference of zero, it is credible. Other differences presented in Tables 8 and 9 can be interpreted similarly.

Tables 10 and 11 give data for 17 diagnostic categories selected for intensive study. Table 10 deals with average number of units of laboratory procedures, by source of payment, while Table 11 shows length of stay evaluation. With respect to construction, the two tables use the models of Tables 8 and 7, respectively, and are to be interpreted similarly.

Comparisons with Estimates from Independent Sources

Whenever data for the universe are available it is enlightening to make comparisons with estimates from the sample. Generally, the number of such comparisons is limited, and for the Michigan study data are available for only two—average length of stay, and number of admissions, the latter being considered comparable with number of discharges. The sample was designed to estimate means or averages well; it was not expected that precise estimates of aggregates would be forthcoming. Data presented in Table 12 demonstrate that the sample performed as designed. Differences between average lengths of stay estimated from the sample and from independent sources range between .1 and .6 days, for all hospitals and by size group. Similar comparisons for aggregate numbers of discharges show substantially more variation. The fact that sample estimates consistently differ from the independent estimates by less than the approximate standard errors may denote overestimation of sampling variability. If this holds generally, then the chances that the true value is included within a range of two standard errors on either side of the sample estimate are greater, by an unknown amount, than 95 in 100.

Because our concept of discharge (or admission) differs from that in use in some large hospitals (500 or more beds), the aggregate number of discharges estimated from the sample is not comparable with number of admissions reported by independent sources; consequently, no comparison is available at the state level.

GENERAL OBSERVATIONS ON THE SAMPLE DESIGN

To express satisfaction with this experience in probability sampling of hospitals and patients is not to imply faultless design or absence of problems. Retrospection suggests alternate procedures to be investigated if sampling is to continue in this subject area. Some exploration of sources of variation preliminary to the Michigan study might have produced an improved sample, but the pressure on time forced a choice between a quickly contrived probability design or a nonprobability selection of hospitals. However, methods acceptable for a one-time study may prove inefficient for repeated or continuing surveys.

For example, it is not certain that number of beds is the best measure of size, nor that the boundaries of hospital size groups as used are to be recommended. Defining size as number of admissions or as average daily census and applying techniques [3, 18, pp. 219–220] available for determining optimum boundaries for size classes may reveal interesting design implications. Some calculations of approximate correlations, by size group, indicate positive but somewhat weak relationships between discharges and number of beds. Furthermore, the sample hospitals show considerable variation among numbers of discharges per bed as indicated by the following:

Hospital size group (number of beds)	Range of numbers of discharges per bed
500 or more	19 to 42
250 to 499	35 to 59
100 to 249	24 to 61
50 to 99	29 to 61
Less than 50	23 to 74

Among sample hospitals there was a tendency for high ratios to be associated with church-operated institutions. In the under-50-bed hospital group the low ratios occurred in populous urban areas and the highest ratios in small community hospitals. Classification by number of admissions may yield more homogeneous groups, with respect to important variables, thus reducing sampling variability.

Motivated by these comments and preliminary examination of the relationships between number of beds and other hospital characteristics, Robert L. Evans, Richard R. Graybeal, and Stephen F. Loebs, students in the Program in Hospital Administration at The University of Michigan, carried out investigations, based on data for the 1958 universe of Michigan general hospitals, that indicate:

1. Even though number of beds shows low correlation with some characteristics considered important to a study of hospitals and patients, it appears to be the best readily available measure for a general, all-purpose study of both patients and institutions.

2. Using number of beds as a measure of size for hospitals with less than 500 beds, and equalizing aggregate number of beds per stratum, the within-group variability of aggregate admissions and of aggregate patient days were reduced about 50 per cent (as compared with the within-group variability for the classifications used in the Michigan study), using six strata defined as:

Stratum	Boundaries (No. of beds)
1	311–499
2	230–310
3	155–229
4	101–154
5	60–100
6	Less than 60

The analysis of variance is presented in Table 13. Questions on an optimum number of strata and their boundaries remain unanswered, however, and deserve further attention. These and other investigations which can be made by using data from current publications [17] and from the Michigan sample will advance the development of optimum sample designs in the field of hospital and medical care.

TABLES 5–13

TABLE 5–Per cent distribution of discharges from general hospitals, and estimated sampling variability of percentages; by diagnostic category, for all hospitals and by size group; State of Michigan, 1958

[Newborn excluded]

Diagnostic Categories [a] (1)	All Hospitals				Group 1 (500 beds and over)				Group 2 (250–499 beds)			
	Est. per cent (2)	Standard error (per cent) (3)	Sample var.[b] srv (4)	No. of sample cases[c] (5)	Est. per cent (6)	Standard error (per cent) (7)	Sample var.[b] srv (8)	No. of sample cases[c] (9)	Est. per cent (10)	Standard error (per cent) (11)	Sample var.[b] srv (12)	No. of sample cases[c] (13)
All Diagnoses	100.0	...	...	9,429	100.0	...	...	1,585	100.0	...	...	2,249
Infective and parasitic diseases [d]	1.3	.16	1.8	98	1.9	.30	.8	23	1.6	.50	3.5	30
Malignant neoplasms [d]	3.0	.22	1.6	218	4.5	.50	.9	55	3.9	.61	2.3	71
Benign and unspecified neoplasms [d]	2.4	.18	1.4	174	2.8	.39	.9	34	2.8	.42	1.5	51
Fibromyomata of uterus	1.1	.07	.4	230	1.3	.05	h	47	1.1	.12	.3	48
Allergic, endocrine, metabolic, etc. [d]	.8	.08	.8	57	1.0	.23	.9	12	.8	.10	.3	15
Asthma	1.0	.06	.4	204	1.0	.14	.3	34	.7	.10	.3	40
Diabetes mellitus	1.1	.06	.4	240	1.2	.21	.6	45	.9	.08	.2	47
Blood and blood-forming organs [d]	.4	.08	1.6	31	.4	g	g	5	.5	g	g	9
Mental, psycho, etc., disorders [d]	1.8	.14	1.0	132	6.6	.43	.5	82	.9	.27	1.8	17
Nervous system and sense organs [d]	4.1	.27	1.8	298	5.4	.53	.9	67	4.9	.82	3.2	90
Diseases of circulatory system [d]	7.2	.34	1.6	526	6.4	.63	1.1	79	7.5	1.04	2.5	137
Acute myocardial infarction	1.1	.06	.4	226	1.2	.17	.4	41	1.1	.09	.2	62
Diseases of respiratory system [d]	5.2	.41	3.2	381	3.9	.96	3.9	48	3.8	.37	.8	69
Bronchopneumonia	2.2	.27	3.3	438	1.3	.10	.1	47	1.7	.20	.6	91
Tonsils and adenoids [d]	6.7	.41	2.5	502	4.1	.57	1.3	54	7.3	.52	.9	133
Diseases of digestive system [d]	6.7	.37	2.0	492	6.2	.48	.6	77	5.7	.70	2.1	104
Appendicitis	2.4	.16	1.1	516	1.5	.12	.2	52	2.2	.24	.6	119
Inguinal hernia	2.1	.09	.4	458	2.1	.14	.2	77	2.6	.12	.1	145
Diarrhoea (under two years)	.8	.06	.4	177	.7	.13	.4	25	.7	.05	.1	40
Cholecystitis and cholelithiasis	1.6	.06	.2	362	1.6	.10	.1	59	1.3	.07	.1	71
Diseases of genito-urinary system [d]	6.3	.40	2.6	465	5.7	.68	1.4	70	6.3	.90	3.1	115
Urinary tract infection	1.6	.11	.8	354	1.4	.15	.3	52	1.2	.20	.8	64
Urinary tract calculus	.9	.06	.4	183	.8	.11	.2	31	.9	.12	.4	47
Conditions of pregnancy •	1.8	.16	1.4	382	1.2	.09	.1	41	1.5	.18	.5	82
Abortion	2.5	.14	.8	542	2.2	.14	.2	81	2.1	.20	.4	115
Delivery [f]	18.7	1.01	6.3	427	12.9	1.08	1.7	52	21.1	1.98	5.3	119
Skin and cellular tissue [d]	1.7	.14	1.1	127	1.9	.30	.8	24	2.0	.28	.9	37
Bones and organs of movement [d]	2.7	.21	1.6	195	3.6	.41	.8	45	2.7	.42	1.5	50
Congenital malformation [d]	.9	.10	1.1	64	2.0	.33	.9	25	1.1	.19	.8	20
Diseases of early infancy [d]	.2	.04	1.1	13	.2	g	g	2	.2	g	g	3
Symptoms, senility, ill-defined cond. [d]	1.8	.21	2.3	130	2.8	.66	2.6	34	1.7	.42	2.4	31
Accidents, poisonings, violence, etc. [d]	6.5	.36	2.0	481	7.9	.46	.5	97	5.9	.70	2.0	109
Fracture of radius and ulna	.6	.04	.3	143	.7	.14	.4	26	.6	.04	.1	32
Fracture of neck of femur	.6	.04	.3	132	.7	.11	.3	28	.6	.05	.1	31
Supp. class for special admissions [d]	.4	.07	1.1	31	1.1	.23	.8	14	.3	g	g	5

Diagnostic Categories [a]	Group 3 (100–249 beds)				Group 4 (50–99 beds)				Groups 5 AND 6 (Less than 50 beds)			
	Est. per cent (14)	Standard error (per cent) (15)	Sample var.[b] srv (16)	No. of sample cases (17)	Est. per cent (18)	Standard error (per cent) (19)	Sample var.[b] srv (20)	No. of sample cases (21)	Est. per cent (22)	Standard error (per cent) (23)	Sample var.[b] srv (24)	No. of sample cases (25)
All Diagnoses	100.0	...	...	2,941	100.0	...	...	1,680	100.0	...	...	974
Infective and parasitic diseases [d]	.9	.21	1.5	20	1.0	.21	.8	12	1.8	.55	1.7	13
Malignant neoplasms [d]	2.4	.33	1.3	56	2.1	.36	1.1	26	1.4	.43	1.3	10
Benign and unspecified neoplasms [d]	2.5	.38	1.8	57	1.3	.32	1.3	16	2.2	.34	.5	16
Fibromyomata of uterus	1.0	.19	1.0	68	1.1	.10	.2	41	1.3	.19	.3	26
Allergic, endocrine, metabolic, etc. [d]	.7	.11	.6	16	.8	.26	1.5	10	.6	g	g	4
Asthma	.9	.09	.3	62	1.2	.23	.8	43	1.2	.21	.4	25
Diabetes mellitus	1.1	.11	.3	76	1.4	.15	.3	44	1.3	.22	.4	28
Blood and blood-forming organs [d]	.5	.19	2.1	12	.3	g	g	4	.1	g	g	1
Mental, psycho, etc., disorders [d]	.8	.18	1.3	18	.8	.29	1.7	10	.7	g	g	5
Nervous system and sense organs [d]	3.8	.39	1.2	89	2.8	.44	1.2	35	2.4	.66	1.9	17
Diseases of circulatory system [d]	7.2	.57	1.4	166	7.8	1.16	3.1	97	6.6	1.13	2.0	47
Acute myocardial infarction	1.1	.15	.6	70	1.0	.07	.1	36	.9	.21	.5	17
Diseases of respiratory system [d]	5.9	.56	1.7	136	7.8	1.38	4.4	97	4.4	1.78	7.4	31
Bronchopneumonia	2.7	.80	7.3	143	2.7	.68	3.0	100	2.6	1.00	3.8	57
Tonsils and adenoids	6.3	.74	3.6	149	7.6	1.26	3.8	95	9.7	1.29	1.9	71
Diseases of digestive system [d]	7.4	.34	2.3	170	8.3	.85	1.6	103	5.4	1.49	4.3	38
Appendicitis	2.4	.20	1.5	163	2.9	.52	1.6	109	3.3	.54	.9	73
Inguinal hernia	1.8	.13	.7	123	1.7	.18	.3	64	2.3	.35	.5	49
Diarrhoea (under two years) [d]	1.0	.13	.5	65	1.0	.14	.3	36	.5	.17	.5	12
Cholecystitis and cholelithiasis	1.5	.22	.3	105	2.2	.22	.4	82	2.1	.07	h	45
Diseases of genito-urinary system [d]	7.2	.89	3.5	167	5.9	.71	1.5	73	5.7	.98	1.8	40
Urinary tract infection	1.7	.22	.8	117	2.2	.28	.6	81	1.8	.57	1.8	40
Urinary tract calculus	.9	.15	.8	58	1.0	.13	.3	35	.5	.13	.3	12
Conditions of pregnancy [e]	2.0	.29	1.3	138	1.7	.36	1.3	63	2.9	.94	3.1	58
Abortion	2.6	.22	.5	183	2.4	.47	1.6	90	3.3	.56	1.0	73
Delivery [f]	20.2	1.74	5.5	144	16.8	1.49	2.7	65	20.4	5.11	15.7	46
Skin and cellular tissue [d]	1.1	.20	1.1	26	1.6	.43	2.0	20	2.8	.46	.8	20
Bones and organs of movement [d]	2.5	.39	1.8	59	1.8	.39	1.4	22	2.7	.98	3.6	19
Congenital malformation [d]	.3	.08	.4	11	.4	g	g	5	.4	g	g	3
Diseases of early infancy [d]	.3	g	g	6	.1	g	g	1	.1	g	g	1
Symptoms, senility, ill-defined cond. [d]	1.3	.24	1.3	30	2.0	.62	3.3	25	1.4	.24	.4	10
Accidents, poisonings, violence, etc. [d]	6.3	.78	3.0	147	6.7	.83	1.8	83	6.2	1.58	4.2	45
Fracture of radius and ulna	.7	.08	.3	45	.7	.08	.2	25	.7	.13	.3	15
Fracture of neck of femur	.5	.07	.3	38	.8	.12	.3	29	.3	g	g	1
Supp. class for special admissions [d]	.4	g	g	8	.2	g	g	3	.1	g	g	6

[a] See APPENDIX for descriptions of the content of each diagnostic category.
[b] The column heading is to be interpreted as sample variance/simple random variance. More specifically, this is sample variance $\sqrt{pq/n}$, where p is the estimated per cent.

$q = 1 - p$, and n is the succeeding column total. To illustrate, the sample size for all diagnoses was 9,429, and the estimated proportion attributed to infective and parasitic diseases was 1.3 per cent with a standard error of .16 per cent (see columns 1, 2 and 3). The approximate variance of the estimate 1.3 is $(.16)^2$ or .0256. The ratio of the sample variance to that of simple random sampling is $.0256 \div \frac{(1.3)(98.7)}{9429}$ or 1.9, which is within rounding error of 1.8 shown in col. 4.

[c] Figures shown are the actual, unweighted numbers of sample cases. A self-weighting sample at the rate of 1 in 48 would have yielded about 22,295 sample cases, the distribution by size group being approximately 3,740, 5,552, 7,024, 3,765 and 2,214 for groups 1 through 5 and 6, respectively.
[d] Numbers of sample cases are a 1 in 3 subsample of the 1 in 48 sample.
[e] Conditions of pregnancy remains a 1 in 48 sample.
[f] Deliveries are a 1 in 10 subsample of the 1 in 48 selection.
NOTE: Categories exclusive of those indicated by d, e, or f were sampled to yield a minimum of three cases per hospital.
[g] Not shown for fewer than 10 sample cases.
[h] Less than .05.

TABLE 6—Estimated average length of stay and approximate sampling variability of estimates, for discharges from general hospitals; by diagnostic category; State of Michigan, 1958

[Newborn excluded]

DIAGNOSTIC CATEGORIES (1)	Estimated average length of stay (in days) (2)	Sampling variability		Number of sample cases in base (5)
		Standard error (in days) (3)	Coefficient of variation (col 3/col. 2) (4)	
All Diagnoses	7.4	.19	.03	9,429
Infective and parasitic diseases	9.1	.86	.09	98
Malignant neoplasms	16.0	1.26	.08	218
Benign and unspecified neoplasms	5.8	.39	.07	174
Fibromyomata of uterus	10.3	.58	.06	230
Allergic, endocrine, metabolic, etc.	7.7	.90	.12	57
Asthma	7.5	.60	.08	204
Diabetes mellitus	12.6	1.23	.10	240
Blood and blood-forming organs	7.7	1.26	.16	31
Mental, psycho., etc. disorders	8.5	.67	.08	132
Nervous system and sense organs	9.8	.92	.09	298
Diseases of circulatory system	10.3	.58	.06	526
Acute myocardial infarction	19.4	.93	.05	226
Diseases of respiratory system	6.7	.37	.06	381
Bronchopneumonia	9.5	.58	.06	438
Tonsils and adenoids	1.7	.12	.07	502
Diseases of digestive system	8.9	.41	.05	492
Appendicitis	6.2	.25	.04	516
Inguinal hernia	7.6	.30	.04	458
Diarrhoea (under two years)	6.0	.42	.07	177
Cholecystitis and cholelithiasis	12.3	.64	.05	362
Diseases of genito-urinary system	7.1	.37	.05	465
Urinary tract infection	7.8	.65	.08	354
Urinary tract calculus	7.7	.59	.08	183
Conditions of pregnancy	2.6	.17	.07	382
Abortion	3.8	.17	.04	542
Delivery	4.8	.16	.03	427
Skin and cellular tissue	8.1	.72	.09	127
Bones and organs of movement	8.9	.60	.07	195
Congenital malformation	11.1	2.29	.21	64
Diseases of early infancy	10.4	3.92	.38	13
Symptoms, senility, and ill-defined cond.	6.1	.47	.08	130
Accidents, poisonings, violence, etc.	6.4	.45	.07	481
Fracture of radius and ulna	4.3	.41	.09	143
Fracture of neck of femur	27.5	2.50	.09	132
Supp. class for special admissions	4.5	.84	.19	31

TABLE 7—Per cent distribution of discharges from general hospitals, and approximate sampling variability of percentages; by primary source of payment[a]; State of Michigan, 1958

[Note: Data relate to the 35 diagnostic categories in Table 5. Newborn are excluded]

PRIMARY SOURCE OF PAYMENT (1)	Estimated per cent (2)	Sampling variability		Number of sample cases[c] (5)
		Standard error (per cent) (3)	Sample var.[b] srv (4)	
All sources	100.0	...	...	9,429
Blue Cross-Blue Shield	50.7	1.97	14.7	4,797
Commercial insurance	21.2	1.37	10.6	2,011
Patient	19.1	.83	4.2	1,700
Other source alone[d]	8.1	.79	7.9	830
All other combinations of sources[e]	.9	.10	1.0	91

[a] "Primary source" categorizes patients according to *principal* contributor to payment of the hospital bill. For example, Blue Cross-Blue Shield includes some cases in which the patient paid a small percentage.

[b] The column heading is to be interpreted as sample variance/simple random variance. See footnote b, Table 5, for additional explanation.

[c] A self-weighting sample at the rate of 1 in 48 would have yielded about 22,295 cases distributed proportionately by source of payment category; the categories do not share proportionately in the sample of 9,429 cases.

[d] Includes welfare, tort action, Medicare, Workmen's Compensation, Armed Forces, Michigan Crippled Children Commission, and other voluntary organizations.,

[e] Includes Blue Cross-Blue Shield *and* commercial insurance, and other similar combinations of payment sources.

TABLE 8—Estimated average total hospital charges, and differences between charges, and approximate sampling variability of estimates; for discharges from general hospitals; by primary source of payment,[a] and by comparison of sources; State of Michigan, 1958

[Note: Data relate to 35 diagnostic categories in Table 5. Newborn are excluded]

CHARACTERISTIC (1)	Average total charges and difference between charges (2)	Sampling variability		Number of sample cases in base (5)
		Standard error (3)	Coefficient of variation (col. 3/col. 2) (4)	
Average total hospital charges, by primary source of payment				
Blue Cross-Blue Shield	$245	$ 8.8	.04	4,797
Commercial insurance	203	7.9	.04	2,011
Patient	222	9.0	.04	1,700
Other source alone[b]	303	19.1	.06	830
All other combinations of sources[c]	301	48.6	.16	91
Difference between average total hospital charges, by comparison of sources				
Blue Cross-Blue Shield vs. commercial insurance	42	10.0	.24	...
Blue Cross-Blue Shield vs. patient	23	10.2	.44	...
Blue Cross-Blue Shield vs. other sources alone[b]	58	20.8	.36	...
Commercial insurance vs. patient	19	9.7	.51	...
Commercial insurance vs. other source alone[b]	100	18.8	.19	...
Patient vs. other source alone[b]	81	20.5	.25	...

[a] "Primary source" categorizes patients according to *principal* contributor to payment of the hospital bill. For example, Blue Cross-Blue Shield includes cases in which the patient paid a small percentage.

[b] Includes welfare, tort action, Medicare, Workmen's Compensation, Armed Forces, Michigan Crippled Children Commission, and other voluntary organizations.

[c] Includes Blue Cross-Blue Shield *and* commercial insurance, and other similar combinations of payment sources.

TABLE 9—Estimated average length of stay, and difference between stays, and approximate sampling variability of estimates; for discharges from general hospitals; by primary source of payment,[a] and by comparison of sources; State of Michigan, 1958

[Note: Data relate to 35 diagnostic categories in Table 5. Newborn are excluded]

CHARACTERISTIC	Average length of stay and difference between stays (in days)	Sampling variability		Number of sample cases in base
		Standard error (in days)	Coefficient of variation (col. 3/col. 2)	
(1)	(2)	(3)	(4)	(5)
Average length of stay, by primary source of payment				
All sources	7.4	0.19	.03	9,429
Blue Cross-Blue Shield	7.4	.21	.03	4,797
Commercial insurance	6.3	.25	.04	2,011
Patient	7.0	.29	.04	1,700
Other source alone[b]	10.5	.43	.04	830
All other combinations of sources[c]	10.2	1.18	.12	91
Difference between average lengths of stay, by comparison of sources				
Blue Cross-Blue Shield vs. commercial insurance	1.1	.25	.23	. . .
Blue Cross-Blue Shield vs. patient	.4	.28	.70	. . .
Blue Cross-Blue Shield vs. other source alone[b]	3.1	.47	.15	. . .
Blue Cross-Blue Shield vs. all sources	[d]	. . .	. . .	. . .
Commercial ins. vs. patient	.7	.30	.43	. . .
Commercial ins. vs. other source alone	4.2	.47	.11	. . .
Commercial ins. vs. all sources	1.1	.18	.16	. . .
Patient vs. other source alone[b]	3.5	.47	.13	. . .
Patient vs. all sources	.4	.22	.55	. . .
Other source alone[b] vs. all sources	3.1	.43	.14	. . .

[a] "Primary source" categorizes patients according to *principal* contributor to payment of the hospital bill. For example, Blue Cross-Blue Shield includes some cases in which the patient paid a small percentage.

[b] Includes welfare, tort action, Medicare, Workmen's Compensation, Armed Forces, Michigan Crippled Children Commission, and other voluntary organizations.

[c] Includes Blue Cross-Blue Shield *and* commercial insurance, and other similar combinations of payment sources.

[d] Less than .05.

TABLE 10—Estimated average number of units of laboratory procedures,[a] and difference between average number of units of procedures; and approximate sampling variability of estimates; for discharges from general hospitals; by primary source of payment,[b] and by comparison of sources; State of Michigan, 1958

[Note: Data relate to 17 diagnoses selected for intensive study]

CHARACTERISTIC	Average number of units of laboratory procedures and difference between units of laboratory procedures	Sampling variability		Number of sample cases in base
		Standard error (in units)	Coefficient of variation (col. 3/col. 2)	
(1)	(2)	(3)	(4)	(5)
Average number of units of laboratory procedures, by primary source of payment				
Blue Cross-Blue Shield	29.6	2.13	.07	2,759
Commercial insurance	23.2	1.50	.06	1,223
Patient	28.1	1.88	.07	1,036
Other source alone[d]	41.8	5.86	.14	454
All other combinations of sources[e]	35.8	12.03	.34	43
Difference between average number of units of laboratory procedures, by comparison of sources				
Blue Cross-Blue Shield vs. commercial	6.4	1.82	.28	...
Blue Cross-Blue Shield vs. patient	1.5	2.41	1.61	...
Blue Cross-Blue Shield vs. other source alone[d]	12.2	6.15	.50	...
Commercial insurance vs. patient	4.9	1.72	.35	...
Commercial insurance vs. other source alone[d]	18.6	5.94	.32	...
Patient vs. other source alone[d]	13.7	6.03	.44	...

[a] Using the results of the Relative Value Study conducted by the Committee on Fees, Commission on Medical Services, California Medical Association, each laboratory procedure for each patient in the intensive study was assigned a weight which roughly reflects the complexity of the procedure. For each hospital stay the weights were added to obtain a composite index of complexity and volume of laboratory procedures. Note that "average number of units" is *not* to be interpreted as average number of procedures.

[b] "Primary source" categorizes patients according to *principal* contributor to payment of the hospital bill. For example, Blue Cross-Blue Shield includes some cases in which the patient paid a small percentage.

[c] See footnote a, Table 11, for diagnoses selected for intensive study.

[d] Includes welfare, tort action, Medicare, Workmen's Compensation, Armed Forces, Michigan Crippled Children Commission, and other voluntary organizations.

[e] Includes Blue Cross-Blue Shield *and* commercial insurance, and other similar combinations of payment sources.

TABLE 11—Per cent distribution of discharges from general hospitals, and approximate sampling variability of percentages; by length of stay evaluation category; State of Michigan, 1958

[Note: Data relate to 17 diagnoses[a] chosen for intensive study]

| | | Sampling variability | | |
| LENGTH OF STAY EVALUATION | Estimated per cent | Standard error (per cent) | Sample var.[b] srv | Number of sample cases[c] |
(1)	(2)	(3)	(4)	(5)
All cases	100.0	. . .	. . .	5,515
Appropriate length of stay	83.1	.95	3.6	4,323
Understay	7.1	.87	6.3	363
Overstay	9.7	.97	5.9	816
Both overstay and understay[d]	.1	.04	.6	13

[a] Fibromyomata of uterus, bronchial asthma, diabetes mellitus, acute myocardial infarction, bronchopneumonia, tonsils and adenoids, appendicitis, inguinal hernia, diarrhoea, cholecystitis and cholelithiasis, urinary tract infection, urinary tract calculus, abortion, delivery, other conditions of pregnancy, fracture of radius and ulna, and fracture of neck of femur. The Effectiveness Study included premature newborn, but they are excluded from the table.

[b] The column heading is to be interpreted as sample variance/simple random variance. See footnote b, Table 5, for additional explanation.

[c] Because the sample was not self-weighting, the length of stay categories do not share proportionately in the base of 5,515 cases. To illustrate, there were 816 overstays in the sample—not 9.7 per cent of 5,515, or 535 cases.

[d] Applies to surgical cases having pre-operative overstay and post-operative understay.

TABLE 12—Comparisons of sample estimates with data from independent source, State of Michigan, 1958

[Data relate to 35 diagnostic categories in Table 5]

CHARACTERISTIC	Sample estimate	Approx. standard error	Data from independent source[a]
Average length of stay in general hospitals (in days)			
All hospitals	7.4	0.2	7.3
Hospitals with 500 or more beds	9.6	0.2	9.8
Hospitals with 250 beds to 499 beds	7.8	b	7.2
Hospitals with 100 beds to 249 beds	6.5	b	6.9
Hospitals with 50 beds to 99 beds	6.8	b	6.7
Hospitals with less than 50 beds	6.0	b	6.3
Number of discharges from general hospitals (in thousands)			
All hospitals	1,070.3	38.8[c]	. . .
Hospitals with 500 or more beds	179.6	1.6	. . .
Hospitals under 500 beds	890.7	38.7	901.5
Hospitals with 250 beds to 499 beds	266.6	25.3	262.3
Hospitals with 100 beds to 249 beds	337.2	32.9	354.4
Hospitals with 50 beds to 99 beds	180.7	22.8	169.0
Hospitals with less than 50 beds	106.3	25.7	115.8

[a] Michigan Hospital Service, Hospital Relations Department, Quarterly Reports, September and December, 1959. Data were unavailable for several of the smaller hospitals (under 25 beds) in the universe. For each of these institutions, the mean number of admissions and average length of stay for the reporting hospitals in the same size group and geographic location were used as estimates.

[b] Standard error not calculated.

[c] The standard errors of estimated discharges from all hospitals, hospitals with 500 or more beds, and hospitals under 500 beds were obtained from the total variance, and the variance components for certainty and noncertainty hospitals, respectively, as defined in equation (7). When calculating standard errors of discharges from the four size groups comprising hospitals under 500 beds, each group was regarded as a separate universe (see Chapter V, footnote 5); hence, the sum of the variances over the four groups is not equivalent to the variance of their sum (that is, the variance for noncertainty hospitals) as defined in equation (7).

TABLE 13—Analysis of variance for two different classifications of Michigan hospitals with less than 500 beds

SOURCE OF VARIATION	FOUR SIZE GROUPS USED IN MICHIGAN STUDY			ALTERNATE GROUPING			COMPARISON OF MEAN SQUARES
	Sum of squares (in millions)	d.f.	Mean square (in millions)	Sum of squares (in millions)	d.f.	Mean square (in millions)	
Patient days							
Total	186,334	223*	...	186,334	223	...	
Between groups	163,638	3	54,546	175,890	5	35,178	$\dfrac{47.9}{103} = .46$
Within groups	22,696	220	103	10,444	218	47.9	
Admissions							
Total	3,435	224*	...	3,435	224	...	
Between groups	2,891	3	963	3,093	5	619	$\dfrac{1.56}{2.46} = .63$
Within groups	544	221	2.46	342	219	1.56	

* Number of admissions was not reported for two hospitals and three did not report number of patient days.

Chapter VI

Summary, Conclusions and Implications

A probability design for a sample of general hospitals and patients is presented and illustrated with a description of a sample of 47 hospitals selected for the Michigan *Study of Hospital and Medical Economics*. Illustrations of worksheets and detailed descriptions of a controlled selection of hospitals are presented for the less technically-oriented person who is interested in utilizing this sampling tool. A controlled subselection of some of the Michigan sample hospitals is also included. Hospital record systems are discussed, sampling techniques are suggested, and formulas for the approximation of sampling variability are provided, along with selected results from the study of the "Character and Effectiveness of Hospital Use."

The technique of controlled selection enables a sampler to reproduce the universe well with a relatively small number of hospitals. The flexibility of design permits supplementation or subsampling of primary (hospitals) or secondary (discharges) selections to meet efficiently the research requirements; on the whole, sampling variability is within limits acceptable for the research needs of the Michigan study.

The Michigan study demonstrates that it is possible to select a probability sample of general hospitals to meet well-defined objectives. In the past, this task has been considered nearly hopeless on the grounds that to be "representative" requires a sample so large that it is almost as practical (or just as impractical) to take the whole universe of hospitals in an area, region, state, or the nation. As a consequence of this judgment, fruitful lines of inquiry have been neglected and approximate answers to research questions have been sought through the collection of broad, general data from all hospitals in a universe. Such data have been useful in many ways, but they could not answer questions in depth or lend themselves to any intensity of exploration.

Depth and intensity have been sought in case studies. Intriguing as these case studies often are, they do more to raise interesting questions than to provide answers. No degree of generalization is possible from them save that found in administrative intuition. The health and hospital fields have need today for sound knowledge rather than intuition alone for the solution of present complex problems and for planning in the face of an uncertain future.

Many new lines of research endeavor can be explored because of the general applicability of conclusions made possible by the use of probability samples of hospitals. A probability sample of patients within a single hospital can be achieved with relative ease. Sampling techniques are highly recommended to replace the time-honored request, "Give me thirty appendectomies." A properly selected sample of patients within a probability sample of hospitals has special significance for clinical and social research. Around this unit—the patient in the hospital—clusters a wealth of retrievable information. It may begin with the medical record and the financial account in the hospital; it extends in a number of directions through the memory, opinions and feelings of the patient himself, his physician and his family. Or, desired information may relate to the administrative and organizational structure of the hospital and its medical staff, and to the functioning of this complex in terms of the input of money, space, equipment, and personnel and the output of diagnostic and therapeutic services. Many different research techniques may be needed to retrieve the useful parts of this mass of information; but these techniques may be employed with the confidence that a measurable degree of precision attaches to the results.

There is no dearth of researchable questions in the hospital field. There is a real and growing need for answers, both on the immediately practical and on the theoretical levels. Because much of the research to supply answers will be conducted on a sample basis, general applicability of these answers depends upon the use of measurable sample designs. If this monograph succeeds in demonstrating the fruitfulness of probability sampling and encourages its use by researchers in the health field, then its primary purpose will be fulfilled.

Selected References

1. Abdellah, F. G., and Levine, E., "Effect of Nurse Staffing on Satisfactions with Nursing Care," *Hospital Monograph Series*, No. 4, Chicago: American Hospital Association, 1958.

2. Cochran, W. G., *Sampling Techniques*. New York: John Wiley and Sons, Inc., 1953.

3. Cochran, W. G., "Comparison of Methods for Determining Stratum Boundaries," *Proceedings of the 32nd Session of the International Statistical Institute*, Tokyo, 1960.

4. Committee on Sampling Techniques in Public Health Statistics, Statistics Section, American Public Health Association, "On the Use of Sampling in the Field of Public Health," *American Journal of Public Health*, 44 (June, 1954), pp. 719–740.

5. Deardorf, N. R., and Frankel, M., *Hospital Discharge Study:* An analysis of 576,623 Patients Discharged from Hospitals in 1933. New York: Welfare Council of New York City, Vol. 1, 1942; Vol. 2, 1943.

6. Deming, W. E., *Some Theory of Sampling*. New York: John Wiley and Sons, Inc., 1950.

7. Deming, W. E., *Sample Design in Business Research*. New York: John Wiley and Sons, Inc., 1960.

8. *Directory of the American Osteopathic Hospital Association*. Davenport, Iowa: American Osteopathic Hospital Association (published annually).

9. Dixon, W. J., and Massey, F. J., *Introduction to Statistical Analysis*, Second Edition. New York: McGraw-Hill, 1957.

10. Fisher, R. A., and Yates, F., *Statistical Tables for Biological, Agricultural and Medical Research* (5th edition). London: Oliver and Boyd, 1957.

11. Fitzpatrick, T. B., Riedel, D. C., and Payne, B. C., "Character and Effectiveness of Hospital Use," in W. J. McNerney, et al., *Study of Hospital and Medical Economics*. To be published by American Hospital Association, Chicago, 1961.

12. Goldstein, M. and Woolsey, T. D., "Hospital Utilization in Saskatchewan with Special Reference to Variation by Size of Hospital." U.S. Department of Health, Education and Welfare, Public Health Service, June, 1955. Processed.

13. Goldstein, M. S., and Woolsey, T. D., "Distance Travelled for Hospital Care in Saskatchewan, 1951." U.S. Department of Health, Education and Welfare, Public Health Service, February, 1956. Processed.

14. Goldstein, M. S., "Morbidity Experience of Saskatchewan General Hospitals, 1951: Frequency and Duration of Hospitalization by Primary Diagnosis." U.S. Department of Health, Education and Welfare, Public Health Service, October, 1958. Processed.

15. Goldstein, M. S., "Multiple Diagnoses of Patients Discharged from Saskatchewan General Hospitals, 1951." U.S. Department of Health, Education and Welfare, Public Health Service, June, 1959. Processed.

16. Goodman, R., and Kish, L., "Controlled Selection—A Technique in Probability Sampling," *Journal of the American Statistical Association*, 45 (September, 1950), pp. 350–372.

17. Guide Issue, *Hospitals*, (Journal of the American Hospital Association; guide issue published annually).

18. Hansen, M. H., Hurwitz, W. H., and Madow, W. G., *Sample Survey Methods and Theory*, Vol. 1. New York: John Wiley and Sons, Inc., 1953.

19. Kendall, M. G., and Buckland, W. R., *A Dictionary of Statistical Terms*. London: Oliver and Boyd, 1957.

20. Kish, L., "Selection of the Sample," in Festinger and Katz (eds.), *Research Methods in the Behavioral Sciences*. New York: Dryden Press, 1953, Chapter 5, pp. 175–239.

21. Kish, L., and Hess, I., "On Variances and Their Differences in Multi-Stage Samples," *Journal of the American Statistical Association*, 54 (June, 1959), pp. 416–446.

22. MacKay, D., "Hospital Morbidity Statistics; a Preliminary Study of In-Patient Discharges," *General Register Office Studies on Medical and Population Subjects*, No. 4, London: His Majesty's Stationery Office, 1951.

23. Madow, L. H., "Systematic Sampling and Its Relation to Other Sampling Designs," *Journal of the American Statistical Association*, 41 (1946), pp. 204–217.

24. New, P. K., Nite, G., and Callahan, J. M., *Nursing Service and Patient Care: A Staffing Experiment*. Kansas City, Missouri: Community Studies, Inc., Publication No. 119, November, 1959.

25. Patton, R. E., "The Sampling of Records," U.S. Department of Health, Education and Welfare, *Public Health Reports*, 67 (October, 1952), pp. 1013–1019.

26. Poland, E., Lembcke, P. A., and Shain, M., *Kansas Nursing Homes:* A Study of Nursing Homes, and Homes for the Aged and Their Patients or Residents. Kansas City, Missouri: Community Studies, Inc., Publication No. 129, November, 1959.

27. Savage, L. J., "Bayesian Statistics," in R. E. Machol and P. Gray (editors), *Decision and Information Processes*. To be published by The Macmillan Co., New York, 1961.

28. Serkin, M. G., Crane, M. M., Brown, M. L., and Kramm, E. R., "A National Hospital Survey of Cystic Fibrosis," U.S. Department of Health, Education and Welfare, *Public Health Reports*, 74 (September, 1959), pp. 764–770.

29. Stephan, F. F., "History of the Uses of Modern Sampling Procedures," *Journal of the American Statistical Association*, 43 (March, 1948), pp. 12–39.

30. Sturdavant, M., et al., "Comparisons of Intensive Nursing Service in a Circular and a Rectangular Unit," *Hospital Monograph Series:* No. 8, Chicago: American Hospital Association, 1960.

31. Winter, K. E., and Metzner, C. A., "Institutional Care for the Long-Term Patient," Bureau of Public Health Economics, *Research Series* No. 7, School of Public Health, The University of Michigan, 1958.

32. Yates, F., *Sampling Methods for Censuses and Surveys* (Second edition). New York: Hafner, 1953.

Appendix

DIAGNOSTIC CATEGORIES EMPLOYED IN THE STUDY OF THE CHARACTER AND EFFECTIVENESS OF HOSPITAL USE AND CORRESPONDING INTERNATIONAL STATISTICAL CLASSIFICATION CODE NUMBERS

I. *Infective and Parasitic Diseases:* 001.0 – 138.0 (excluding: 016.1 tuberculosis, kidney; 016.2 tuberculosis, other urinary)
001.0 – 008.0 Tuberculosis of respiratory system
010.0 – 019.2 Tuberculosis, other forms (excluding: 016.1 and 016.2)
020.0 – 029.0 Syphilis and its sequelae
030.0 – 039.0 Gonococcal infection and other venereal diseases
040.0 – 049.0 Infectious disease commonly arising in intestinal tract
050.0 – 064.4 Other bacterial diseases
070.0 – 074.1 Spirochaetal diseases, except syphilis
080.0 – 096.9 Diseases attributable to viruses
100.0 – 108.0 Typhus and other rickettsial diseases
110.0 – 117.0 Malaria
120.0 – 138.0 Other infective and parasitic diseases

II. *Malignant Neoplasms:* 140.0 – 205.0
140.0 – 148.0 Malignant neoplasm of buccal cavity and pharynx
150.0 – 159.0 Malignant neoplasm of digestive organs and peritoneum
160.0 – 165.9 Malignant neoplasm of respiratory system
170.0 – 181.7 Malignant neoplasm of breast and genito-urinary organs
190.0 – 199.8 Malignant neoplasm of other and unspecified sites
200.0 – 205.0 Neoplasms of lymphatic and haematopoietic tissues

III. *Benign and Unspecified Neoplasms:* 210.0 – 239.0 (excluding: 214.0 uterine fibromyoma)
210.0 – 229.0 Benign neoplasms (excluding 214.0)
230.0 – 239.0 Neoplasms of unspecified nature

IV. *Uterine Fibromyoma:* 214.0

V. *Allergic, Endocrine System, Metabolic, and Nutritional Diseases:* 240.0 – 289.3 (excluding: 241.0 asthma; 260.0 – 260.9 diabetes mellitus)
240.0 – 245.3 Allergic disorders (excluding 241.0)
250.0 – 254.1 Diseases of thyroid gland
270.0 – 277.2 Diseases of other endocrine glands
280.0 – 289.3 Avitaminoses and other metabolic diseases

VI. *Asthma:* 241.0

VII. *Diabetes Mellitus:* 260.0 – 260.9

VIII. *Diseases of the Blood and Blood-Forming Organs:* 290.0 – 299.0

IX. *Mental, Psychoneurotic, and Personality Disorders:* 300.0 – 329.9
300.0 – 309.2 Psychoses
310.0 – 319.9 Psychoneurotic disorders
320.0 – 329.9 Disorders of character, behavior and intelligence

X. *Diseases of the Nervous System and Sense Organs:* 330.0 – 398.3
330.0 – 334.1 Vascular lesions affecting central nervous system
340.0 – 345.0 Inflammatory diseases of central nervous system
350.0 – 357.0 Other diseases of central nervous system
360.0 – 369.0 Diseases of nerves and peripheral ganglia
370.0 – 379.0 Inflammatory diseases of eye
380.0 – 389.3 Other diseases and conditions of eye
390.0 – 398.3 Diseases of ear and mastoid

XI. *Diseases of the Circulatory System:* 400.0 – 468.3 (excluding: 420.3 acute myocardial infarction)

    400.0 – 402.1 Rheumatic fever
    410.0 – 416.0 Chronic rheumatic heart disease
    420.0 – 422.2 Arteriosclerotic and degenerative heart disease (excluding 420.3)
    430.0 – 434.8 Other diseases of heart
    440.0 – 443.0 Hypertensive heart disease
    444.0 – 447.0 Other hypertensive disease
    450.0 – 456.3 Disease of the arteries
    460.0 – 468.3 Diseases of veins and other diseases of circulatory system

XII. *Acute Myocardial Infarction:* 420.3

XIII. *Diseases of the Respiratory System:* 470.0 – 527.2 (excluding: 491.0 bronchopneumonia; 510.0 hypertrophy of tonsils and adenoids)

    470.0 – 475.0 Acute upper respiratory infections
    480.0 – 483.0 Influenza
    490.0 – 493.4 Pneumonia (excluding 491.0)
    500.0 – 502.1 Bronchitis
    510.0 – 527.2 Other diseases of respiratory system (excluding 510.0)

XIV. *Bronchopneumoia:* 491.0

XV. *Tonsils and Adenoids:* 510.0

XVI. *Diseases of the Digestive System:* 530.0 – 587.3 (excluding: 550.0 – 552.2 appendicitis; 560.0 and 561.0 inguinal hernia; 571.0* diarrhoea under two years; 584.0 and 585.0 cholecystitis and cholelithiasis)

    530.0 – 539.4 Diseases of buccal cavity and esophagus
    540.0 – 545.3 Diseases of stomach and duodenum
    550.0 – 553.0 Appendicitis (excluding 550.0 – 552.2)
    560.0 – 561.6 Hernia of abdominal cavity (excluding 560.0 and 561.0)
    570.0 – 578.5 Other diseases of intestines and peritoneum (excluding 571.0*)
    580.0 – 587.3 Diseases of liver, gallbladder, and pancreas (excluding 584.0 and 585.0)

XVII. *Appendicitis:* 550.0 – 552.2

XVIII. *Inguinal Hernia:* 560.0 and 561.0

XIX. *Diarrhoea under two years of age:* 571.0*

XX. *Cholecystitis and Cholelithiasis:* 584.0 and 585.0

XXI. *Diseases of the Genito-Urinary System:* 016.1, 016.2, 590. – 637.6 (excluding: 016.1, 016.2, 600.0, 603.0, 605.0, 606.0, 609.0 and 609.3 urinary tract infections; 602.0 and 604.0 urinary tract calculus)

    590.0 – 594.0 Nephritis and nephrosis
    600.0 – 609.3 Other diseases of urinary system (excluding 600.0, 603.0, 605.0, 606.0, 609.0 609.3, 602.0 and 604.0)
    610.0 – 617.3 Diseases of male genital organs
    620.0 – 626.3 Diseases of breast, ovary, Fallopian tube, and parametrium
    630.0 – 637.6 Diseases of uterus and other female organs

XXII. *Urinary Tract Infections:* 016.1, 016.2, 600.0, 603.0, 605.0, 606.0, 607.0, 609.0, 609.3

XXIII. *Urinary Tract Calculus:* 602.0 and 604.0

XXIV. *Conditions and Complications of Pregnancy, Childbirth, and the Puerperium:* 640.0 – 688.6 (excluding: 648.0, 648.5, 650 – 652.3 abortion; 660.0 – 678.3 delivery)

    640.0 – 649.0 Complications of pregnancy (excluding 648.0, 648.5)
    680.0 – 688.6 Complications of the puerperium

XXV. *Abortion:* 648.0, 648.5, 650.0 – 652.3

XXVI. *Delivery:* 660.0 – 678.3

XXVII. *Diseases of the Skin and Cellular Tissue:* 690.0 – 716.1

    690.0 – 698.1 Infections of skin and cellular tissue
    700.0 – 716.1 Other diseases of skin and subcutaneous tissue

XXVIII.   *Diseases of the Bones and Organs of Movement:* 720.0 – 749.9
      720.0 – 727.0 Arthritis and rheumatism, except rheumatic fever
      730.0 – 738.9 Osteomyelitis and other disease of bone and joint
      740.0 – 749.9 Other diseases of musculoskeletal system

XXIX.   *Congenital Malformations:* 750.0 – 759.3

XXX.   *Diseases of Early Infancy:* 760.0 – 776.0
      760.0 – 769.9 Birth injuries, asphyxia, and infections of newborn
      770.0 – 776.0 Other diseases peculiar to early infancy

XXXI.   *Symptoms, Senility, and Ill-Defined Conditions:* 780.0 – 795.6
      780.0 – 789.8 Symptoms referable to systems or organs
      790.0 – 795.6 Senility and ill-defined diseases

XXXII.   *Accidents, Poisonings, Violence, Nature of Injury:* 800.0 – 999.9 (excluding: 813.0 –813.2†
                                                             fracture radius and ulna; 820.0 – 820.2
                                                             fracture neck of femur)
      800.0 – 809.9 Fracture of skull, spine and trunk
      810.0 – 819.9 Fracture of upper limb (excluding 813.0 – 813.2)
      820.0 - 829.9 Fracture of lower limb (excluding 820.0 – 820.2)

XXXIII.   *Fracture of Radius and Ulna:* 813.0 – 813.2†

XXXIV.   *Fracture of Neck of Femur:* 820.0 – 820.2

XXXV.   *Supplementary Classifications for Special Admissions:* y00.0 – y18.0
      y00.0 – y09.2 Special conditions and examination without sickness
      y10.0 – y18.0 Admissions for convalescent care, plastic treatment, and fitting
                 of prosthetic device.

---

* 571.1   Diarrhoea over two years of age
† 818.0   Fracture of radius alone included in general category XXXII: Accidents, Poisonings, etc.